This book is for you if you...

- want to make a difference in maternity services and advocate for woman-centred and person-centred care

- feel frustrated with the current state of maternity care and want to learn how to instigate change

- are a parent or expectant mother looking for insights on navigating maternity care effectively

- are a midwife or birth worker seeking practical strategies to support your clients and improve services

- are part of a community group or organisation focused on maternity issues and want to strengthen your impact and campaigns

- are interested in activism and want to understand the journey of a seasoned campaigner in the maternity sector

- want to learn from real experiences and gain actionable advice on how to campaign for better maternity services

- believe in the power of collective action and want to be inspired by stories of successful campaigns and activism

"As a life enters and leaves this world, it is precious. Those moments are precious and fragile and need to be held in total love and respect. Ruth Weston passionately advocates this with regards to birth and those that support it – mothers and midwives. I resonate deeply as one of my babies, deceased at four months, was failed by the system, during a birth and a period after of pure hell.

Born Stroppy packs a powerful, honest, brave punch of reality and love. It's a wake-up and a shake-up to something that really, really matters and that is so overlooked."

Jacky Seery
Mindfulness Teacher | Qigong and Yoga Teacher |
Soul Midwife | Owner of Mind Body One

***

"*Born Stroppy* is a rich patchwork, carefully sewn together, with very different panels, which will be of use to birth activists and others working around women's health. Different readers will find their own gems within the overall pattern.

As well as honestly telling the story of her own activism, including burnout and breakdown, Ruth Weston looks at strategies, tools and tactics for bringing about change. The analysis of ways to work against an oppressive system was a gem I found useful for myself and as a way of understanding the differing reactions of others to the crisis in maternity services.

There are reflection points and suggestions for practices which are succinct and useful. There is a lot of wisdom, and

Ruth draws upon different spiritual traditions, a great deal of heartfelt common sense and her awareness that 'activism has to be energising for it to be sustainable'. *Born Stroppy* is vital reading for anyone who cares about the future of maternity services."

Mavis Kirkham
Emeritus Professor of Midwifery at
Sheffield Hallam University | Author of *Informed Choice in Maternity Care, Birth Centres: A social model of maternity care, The Midwife/Mother Relationship,* and *Exploring the Dirty Side of Women's Health.*

***

"Ruth is a trained liberation theologian, a community organiser and a birth activist, with intensive experience of living in deprived areas such as Bradford. I have been privileged to read early drafts of her remarkable and stimulating book, *Born Stroppy,* which is part autobiography, part activist manual, part spiritual journal; through it, she provides a remarkable insight into a mature, creative activism that is beyond cynicism.

Although this is a book about childbirth in contemporary Britain and the struggles of mothers – and needs to be read by anyone involved in midwifery – it is germane to all those who see themselves as activists in totally different arenas. Ruth offers stories of real women, not least herself, and the tribulations of having a birth in the way that you want. Through it all, we see someone taking themselves and their concerns and their struggles with officialdom seriously and taking creative action as a consequence; the strategic activism of trying to get things done in a difficult, complicated and compromised world. Passing on her learning, experience and skills developed over many years, anyone and everyone can learn from Ruth's hard-won wisdom. Here is a mother and activist who should be taken seriously because she speaks with authentic authority, whatever the authorities might think.

Buy it. Read it. Let it change how you see yourself and how you act in the world."

Revd Dr Ian K Duffield

Director of Research, Urban Theology Union | Doctoral Supervisor with Luther King Centre and the University of Manchester | Author and Contributor to various journals including *Theology* and *The Expository Times*

***

"I love *Born Stroppy*. It helps make sense of my own journey and affirms a lot of what I have learned. I am so pleased Ruth Weston wrote it as it fills a gap in the world of maternity activism."

Deborah Hughes

Midwife | Mother | Veteran Campaigner for woman-led care and true midwifery

***

"*Born Stroppy* is humbling, fury-inducing, immensely useful as a toolkit, and deeply inspiring – especially in how to advocate for the others suffering trauma while healing your own health.

It is an incredible eye-opening account of Ruth Weston's 30+ years of grassroots activism which has truly improved maternity care and knowledge of the birth rights for thousands of women, babies and communities. It is also an extremely practical toolkit for maternity activism, breaking advocacy and activism down into different component parts, and offering a wealth of clear, practical tips, illustrated with realistic examples on how to challenge, disrupt, press for transparency, and drive systemic change at every level of local to national activism. These are suggestions, strategies and tools that will take ordinary, frustrated people from overwhelm at the huge issues in the system, to confident agitator for their own rights and for those of their family and community.

For the absolute beginner campaigner, the chapters on finding your allies and on media and social media are brilliant, practical usable guidance. The structural injustice Ruth describes is held up to the light and robustly criticised for its inequity. *Born Stroppy* also brilliantly explains the systemic harm from misogyny, sexism, patriarchy and racism too, and in the socio-historical context.

This book will not be pigeon-holed! It is part memoir, part history of the birth activism in Yorkshire for over 25 years, part incredibly powerful toolkit for activism, partly a call to remember the vitalness of who we are, and part offering ways to sustain our own souls and mental health when fighting the most harmful systems. *Born Stroppy* is ALL these things with the constant compass running through it of all of Ruth's steadfast, true values.

It has been a beautiful way to spend an afternoon reading Ruth's 'herstory' and deep wisdom."

Jo Rhys-Davies
Human Rights Law Advocate | Barrister (Retired) |
Co-founder of Airedale Mums

***

"Ruth Weston is brilliant, brave and bloody-minded – her passion and intelligence come through so loudly. Her voice is clear, reflective, honest and full of humour. I recommend *Born Stroppy* to anyone involved in maternity care who cares about the experiences women and babies have.

This book comes as a timely call to action, a reminder that our work here is not done, and that we need to reinvigorate birth activism to improve care for women and babies. Maternity services in the UK increasingly focus on pathology, risk and medicalisation, instead of health promotion, resulting in increased maternal morbidity due to excessive levels of interventions.

Some of us may feel fatigued or despondent that our efforts over decades to challenge a system that seems locked on a course it is unwilling to alter, have come to so little. However, Ruth's optimism, experience and know-how is what is needed to re-energise and refocus us. We must challenge a maternity system where standardised rather than individualised care is given, where clinical opinion can trump evidence, where fragmented care persists, and where women are rarely supported to make informed choices.

Ruth's story intertwines with mine and it is painful to be reminded of all the times I witnessed care that was lacking, supported women who felt let down and broken by the system, and how our attempts to change things for the better were often stymied. It is time again to rally and campaign for better maternity care in the UK.

I hope *Born Stroppy* will inspire people to get active!"

Dr Michelle Irving
Midwifery Lecturer | Former Independent Midwife |
Founder of Best Births

***

"Public involvement in how services are run, indeed how the country is run, is vital. Ruth Weston shows what she's achieved as a campaigner and learned along the way. An inspiring book on things we can all do to shape our communities and work towards making the world a better place."

Mary Newburn
Patient and Public Involvement and Engagement Lead
at Mary Newburn Consulting / King's College London
ARC Maternity & PMH theme

***

"*Born Stroppy* is fantastic – both inspiring and thought-provoking. After her long career as a birth activist, Ruth Weston speaks of now aspiring to be 'a granny in the kitchen', one who supports and nurtures those on the front line. 'Grannies', of course, are also the holders of hard-won wisdom from which the next generation would do well learn.

This is what she does so well in this inspiring and thought-provoking book – passing on the lessons from her own journey through birth activism, with characteristic humour and insight, to those who are ready to step forward and find their own ways to make change happen. Anyone who is concerned about the state of our maternity services and wants to do something about it, whether at local or national level, should read this book."

Nadia Higson

AIMS Trustee, Coordinator and Campaigns Volunteer

***

"What sets *Born Stroppy* apart, and takes it beyond a series of engaging and necessary guides in building an effective campaign, is the deeply personal and autobiographical thread that runs seamlessly throughout, holding the many disparate concepts together. After all, the personal is political.

Ruth Weston's life and experiences as an activist leading the campaign for change in the maternity system in the UK – alongside being a mother of five children, a social entrepreneur and small business owner – are gripping.

Each experience is hard-won and gives immense weight to Ruth's guidance. At one point, I was crying; at another, I was laughing; and at another, I was taking notes. When my physical copy arrives, I will very likely be underlining and tabbing pages too!

Born Stroppy is generous, informed and thoughtful. It is written about and aimed in general at those engaging with maternity services and systems in the UK, but offers the reader so much more, and there are takeaways for anyone wanting to make a difference, no matter how small."

Hannah Alwan-Weston
Mum-to-be

***

"I love how Ruth Weston's writing takes you on such a journey but with a dose of fun and tongue-in-cheek. Her determination and drive to make birth better for so many was so inspiring. I raced through *Born Stroppy*, totally ignoring all around me as I was so engrossed!

Anyone who thinks 'I want to change things but one person can't make change,' should read this book. Activists are the core of society and from small acorns, oak trees grow.

Caz Sayles
Doula and Advocate for Birthing Rights

***

"I was delighted when I heard that Ruth Weston was writing a book that would include reflections on her time as a birth activist. Ruth was a welcome – and welcoming – fellow traveller in the 'service user division' of the maternity service improvement community when I first got involved with this work. We overlapped for just a few years, before Ruth sadly felt the need to step back as her activist burnout grew stronger. But these were good years. I witnessed Ruth's determination to make a difference, and the joy she took from working on key issues and delivering inspiring speeches. I looked forward to reading more about Ruth's work and activist philosophy, and this book certainly delivers."

Jo Dagustun
AIMS Volunteer

***

"Changing the world of birth means giving those with the passion for activism the tools to take the plunge. Who better to share these tools than the woman who has been at the leading edge of change in birth activism for over two decades? Ruth Weston shares her life experience as an activist who makes things happen, who gets things done. Anyone, lay or professional, who is interested in making birth better, needs *Born Stroppy*!"

Emma Ashworth
Birth Rights Consultant and Activist,
Former Trustee of AIMS

***

"There is an august tradition of grassroots activism. From Rosa Parks to Greta Thunberg, when women rise and resist, things change. But without people like Ruth Weston, who work to pass down the learning from that activism, we are lost. It is not enough to speak truth to power: the next generation need the tools. *Born Stroppy* is part memoir, part handbook; an engaging instruction manual for women and birthing people everywhere who are being handed the baton. This ship will not be turned in our lifetime, so this book will serve as a record of what works, and a map for our onward journey. Thank you, Ruth."

Maddie McMahon

Doula, Owner of Developing Doulas, and Author of
Why Doulas Matter and *Why Mothering Matters*

***

"*Born Stroppy* is an absolute roller coaster of a book! One minute, I was up in arms; the next minute, sobbing! Ruth's book is a 'warts and all' picture of the state of maternity care in the UK and how little has changed in 60-odd years.

Born Stroppy has an immediacy and dynamism that makes the reader sit up and take notice – this is no passive read! Some passages are brutal and upsetting whilst others are uplifting and make the reader feel like they can overcome anything with the author at their side. It is thought-provoking and instructive, and gives a voice to the thousands of women who don't 'want to make a fuss', who are quashed, silenced and ignored. "

Olivia Eisinger
Editor | Mother

For Midwives, Doulas and Parents

Born Stroppy

Make Change Happen!

Amy,

Have courage and be inspired

You know where I am

if you want a chat

[signature]

May 2025

Ruth Weston

First published in Great Britain in 2025
by Book Brilliance Publishing
265A Fir Tree Road, Epsom, Surrey, KT17 3LF
United Kingdom
+44 (0)20 8641 5090
www.bookbrilliancepublishing.com
admin@bookbrilliancepublishing.com

A CIP catalogue record for this book is
available at the British Library.

ISBN 978-1-913770-97-6

To the women on whose shoulders I stand on,
with gratitude for your inspiration, courage and wisdom.
Without your battles and insight,
we could not have made it this far.

For the sisters and siblings who I have worked alongside,
with gratitude for your love and support, inspiration
and determination. I could not have done this without you.

For the women who stand on my shoulders:
reach for the stars, sisters, and go beyond our dreams.
We are with you every step of the way.

Contents

Foreword

I HAVE KNOWN RUTH Weston for many years, our paths crossing at maternity events from time to time. I hold Ruth in high regard as a woman who has not only lived her own inadequate experiences of childbearing, but as someone who has called out poorly performing maternity services.

For my own part, I have probably walked the same path as Ruth. However, I was a midwife *inside* maternity services striving for change and, more importantly, to uphold the sanctity of childbearing. I was introduced to the visionary GP Dr Luke Zander, who founded the Maternity and Newborn Forum, hosted by the Royal Society of Medicine. Luke was, and probably still is, an activist in the birth world. He challenged the sweeping measures put in place during the late 1960s and 70s of all women birthing in hospital. I was a very new midwife in the early 80s and heard him speak.

His view was, *"Since there is no evidence that home is less safe than hospital, the provision of support for home birth seems not only fully justifiable, but mandatory"*.[1] (Savage, W 1996). And even though we now have irrefutable evidence about where to birth, maternity services still seem unable to implement a reversal of all women birthing in hospital.

Personal is always political in my book. So, it was frustrating to see that in 2024 two female MPs in the House of Commons spoke so negatively yet powerfully of the trauma they had endured during their own recent childbearing. Then followed an enquiry into birth trauma, which was published and reported back to the House of Commons in May 2024[2]. Forgive me for being cynical, but I have been speaking about women's mental health and trauma from maternity and its impact upon families since the late 1990s. But it takes someone from outside of the system to raise concerns.

Likewise with miscarriage. Ruth writes about her own experiences in this arena; the inhumane treatment that women and their partners are forced to endure when they lose their baby. I remember being told by a senior midwife to take the stillborn or miscarried baby away to the sluice quickly so that the woman could not see her infant. God forbid any woman who asked to see her baby before it was taken; these poor women were castigated and often treated appallingly. Their grief was further complicated by the system's attitude to birth and death. Things certainly had to change – does it really have to take more than my 43 years in midwifery to see that?

Lately we have witnessed expensive investigation after investigation, report after report, government-led review after review, speaking to thousands of women, families and clinicians. Yet we are no further forward in the quest for a kind, considerate and respectful birth where women are given real choice and are listened to. The money that all these reports have cost is astronomical and yet maternity services continue to herd women into systems that are broken. Complaints and legal redress is now commonplace and there is probably no maternity unit in the UK that can honestly stand up and say they are offering a service that is completely woman- and family-focused.

Ruth's lifetime of calling for change – with many hours of banging on doors to be heard and never deviating – is admirable and has probably cost her health. In *Born Stroppy*, she is asking all of us to wake up and insist on changes to maternity services that women deserve.

Ruth has documented strategies and given advice on tactics that have worked, and has given much credit to those who have stood beside her along the way. As a midwife, I have worked hard from the inside to change and influence people and services. The reality is that consistent change is only achieved when women and their partners force the issue and shout loudly about what is not acceptable.

I urge birth workers, midwives, doctors and service providers to read this book and examine the care that is delivered in their own establishments. It will be the only way that meaningful change is achieved. If we do not treat women kindly in their most vulnerable hour, then what does that say about us?

Too many birth activists are ageing and tiring of their cause célèbre; it is now up to women and families to open the way for better and compassionate maternity care. Ruth is not unique in her quest for a better childbirth experience;

however, she has taken the precious time and effort to document her journey and that makes her very special.

I am blessed to have known and spent time with Ruth, I am now privileged to invite you all to take the baton she has so steadfastly held.

Dr Kathryn Gutteridge

RM SRN Dip; MSc Counselling & Psychotherapy, Dr Science, Former President Royal College Midwives

A Note About Language

INCLUSIVE LANGUAGE and what it means has become a controversial and polarising debate within maternity in recent years. With this in mind, I want to be clear about the language used in this book and the thinking behind it.

In my view, women – particularly women who are within the maternity system, including mothers, midwives, doulas and indeed female obstetricians – are part of an oppressed group subject to the historical and current ravages of patriarchy and discrimination. Amongst this group, women of colour suffer more greatly than white educated feminists, such as myself. This history(s) and the impact it has on our current predicament should not be underestimated, devalued or denied by anyone.

By the same token, LGBTQ+ people and, particularly within the current controversy, trans people, also have their own history of oppression and discrimination which impacts their current experience and how they are treated and spoken of in our culture. This systemic reality, which is indeed another facet of our patriarchy, cannot and should not denied or underestimated.

What I wish to state clearly is that these two realities are not in competition, and there should be no hierarchy of oppression: they stem from the same culture of 'othering' people who are not cis male or white. Although our histories and experience of discrimination differ, we share the same pain of not being 'seen' and our experience and knowledge not being validated.

The use of language has become the fault line for feminists and gender activists in maternity – one side wanting to ensure they remain visible, the other seeking visibility within the maternity system. Both objectives are valid. Where there is conflict is where the language requirements of one impinge on the language requirements of the other, and this has become distressing for all sides. From my point of view, the conflict tragically detracts energy and focus from the elephant in the room which is the ongoing systemic oppression of all birthing women and people, doulas and midwives, which is having lasting negative physical and psychological impacts on us all, especially our children.

My request is that we seek to understand and accommodate the history, pain and requirements of each other where we can, and to tolerate our differences where we cannot. In this scenario, we simultaneously hold with respect and acceptance two perspectives of historical discrimination, two contrasting experiences, cultures and languages, being willing to hold the dissonance of contradicting demands and understanding, because in alliance we have a bigger enemy to beat in the systemic discrimination and oppression which is the reality of us all.

With this in mind, I have sought to use the new conventions of additional language: 'women' and 'birthing people'.

However, I also sometimes choose to use the words 'mothering' and 'mother' as non-gender-specific terms that also retain the weight of historical gender discrimination, enabling two realities to be recognised at once. This is already recognised in the terms 'midwife' and 'midwifery', non-gendered terms which while encompassing the reality of other genders as midwives, also holds within it the historic structural cultural and socio-economic discrimination that midwives have suffered as a result of it being work overwhelmingly done by women and for women.

There are two areas where, I would argue, this has already been the case for a number of years and where this definition of the term is rooted.

As a progressive Church in the 1990s, we struggled with how to handle 'Mothering Sunday'. Over a period of years, we moved from celebrating only biological and adoptive mothers, to celebrating all women in the Church, whether mothers or not, to celebrating all those 'who mother' of whatever gender, orientation, age or role. This latter understanding of 'mothering' and the role of a mother incorporated all those who fulfilled a mothering role for a child, and encompassed grandparents who provided childcare, parents of both genders, teachers, social and care workers, and also those who provided a caring role to elders in their family and community.

What we found ourselves recognising as a Church community was the usually unacknowledged and invisible care work that goes on in our communities, often perceived as 'women's work', usually, but not exclusively, undertaken by women and so historically subjected to lower status, lower visibility and discrimination. In doing this, we both acknowledged the inclusivity of the role across all genders and sexualities in reality, whilst recognising the systemic gender-specific discrimination that underlies the term as well. I think this is the right way to go.

Secondly, in the Majority South[3] where children have lost their biological mothers and parents due to famine, disease and war, fathers and grandparents have taken over the full role of mother, with stories of grandmothers and fathers lactating to provide sustenance to young orphans. Once again this demonstrates the expansiveness and flexibility of the mothering role in reality whilst retaining the historical and social contexts that are important in tackling discrimination.

In these two contrasting situations, the concept of 'mother' has been expanded to be inclusive of women and people who give birth, and also those of whatever gender or age who fulfil that role. At the same time, we also acknowledge the gender-specific discrimination that is also inherent in the term. This is the inclusivity that I will be using when I employ the term, and I hope this is acceptable to readers and where it is not, that it will be tolerated with the recognition of the heart of inclusivity that beats behind it.

I hope it goes without saying that in a client/pastoral/personal relationship that the words used with the person or couple will be those they choose for themselves. The compassionate holding of different lived realities and perspectives enables us to employ different terms according to the circumstances.

In Chapter 9 (and in the conclusion where it pertains to Chapter 9) and at other points, however, I have retained the full feminine and feminist language as I critique the current outcomes of historic systemic discrimination against all those who identify as women. I am unapologetic of this language as I am unapologetic of my critique of attitudes and policy that hobble the equality and respect of women in the maternity sector.

If this does not reflect your experience or understanding then it probably is not your problem; give thanks and move on: this is a book that is written from one activist's perspective and I recognise therefore that it will not cover the experience of everyone.

At the same time, many folk believe it is only they that experience such problems and see it therefore as personal failure, when in actual fact it is systemic sexism playing out in our own lives.

I hope those who do not share these problems will stand in solidarity with those of us who do, as we will stand in solidarity with you in your challenges.

Together, we will overcome.

Ruth Weston

October 2024

Introduction

I AM A BIRTH ACTIVIST because I want the birth culture of the UK to be woman- and person-centred, not system-centred, and I want my children to receive the care from the NHS that we did not.

I am the mother of five children. I booked five home births, four with the NHS; of these, one transferred in for slow progress, one transferred in after birth for blood loss, and two were normal home water births. The fifth child was born at home under the care of an independent midwife.

I am a theologian specialising in the practice of theologies of liberation. Theologies of liberation are part of the family of theologies and movements of liberation and empowerment that include Black theology, womanist theology, anti-apartheid movements, feminist, LGBTQ+ and disability liberation and rights movements. I am a veteran of the Urban Theology Union in Sheffield. I am a community organiser specialising in building networks, change-making and setting things up or turning things around. And as a change-maker, on impulse, I became the owner of Aquabirths

Birthing Pools in order to ensure birth pools were available to northern women at prices they could afford. We now make beautiful quality birth pools for hospitals in the UK and abroad. I was Chair of Bradford and Airedale MSLC (Maternity Services Liaison Committee), the stakeholder committee for maternity services for Bradford district, stepping down in 2013.

In 2003, with a kind stranger holding my six-month-old, I had a standing ovation for a speech to the Association for the Improvement of Maternity Services (AIMS) and the Association of Radical Midwives (ARM) Conference in Birmingham. In a sense, it is where my book began, when I started to speak out loudly and in public about changing the maternity system and calling it to account. And because things have not substantially changed since then and the questions I asked have still not been answered, here is the start of the speech. Please note that this is an unedited quote from 2003 and I would use different terms now.

It was my first baby. I had booked a home birth but had been transferred after 18 hours for lack of progress and possible meconium. In hospital I had been put on a drip and suffered agonies without any pain relief.

All of a sudden, at the darkest hour I felt it… it was like a pop inside, my contractions felt different and I felt that maybe this baby was going to be born!

The midwife was summoned. "I think I want to push," I told her. I was examined.

"You are 10 cm," she said. "But let a doctor check you."

I was surprised and asked, "Where is the doctor? When will he be here?"

"In about 15 minutes," came the reply.

I said to the midwife, "I have waited 24 hours to have this baby. I am not waiting any longer. You are a midwife! Do your job!" However, I did not say it quite as politely as that!

This little cameo encapsulates much of what I want to say about what needs to change in the birthing care women receive today.

In the UK, we do not have woman-centred care: we have consultant-centred care. Woman-centred care is where the care revolves around the woman and her wants, needs and foibles. Woman-centred care is based on mutual respect and open access to information; the woman speaks directly to the professionals who control her care, and these professionals will refer the woman to specialists if and when this may be needed.

With consultant-centred care, a doctor who you may never see, or a committee of professionals where you have no representation, dictates the choices you can make for birth. In many institutions, the consultant is still at the top of the hierarchy, the centre of the wheel. The service women receive revolves around their interests and their wants, needs and foibles.

The needs and wants of the birthing woman are subjugated by a system that puts the medical practitioner at the centre. For example, Bradford's birthing pool was in the basement for 13 years, not because women did not want it – they were never asked – but because the head consultant was totally against water births. His exact words to me were, "Only whales and dolphins have babies under water."

Consultants specialise in abnormal birth. They are skilled in dealing with the medical problems that may occur in pregnancy and birth, and they save lives – and we are grateful for that. However, we resent the way in which this has been done; taking away our autonomy as women, the professional independence of midwives, and exerting authority over normal birthing which is outside their specialism. For example: in Bradford, rather than midwives, who are the experts in physiological birth, deciding on the merits of birthing pools as pain relief in physiological births, it was the specialists in abnormal birth, the consultants who made the decision.

And so in 1998, a senior midwife visited me at home and we both had to sign something to say that she had told me what a 'bad' choice I had made to choose warm water for my pain relief at my second birth. And so there I was at home, 8 cm dilated and in transition, when one of the midwives announced, "At this moment, I have to ask you to leave the pool as it is not Bradford Trust's policy to allow you to remain in the pool for the birth." Imagine! I politely refused and proceeded to give birth in the pool unimpeded – but what a farce! So even though the consultant was not present at my NHS births, he was present in the actions of the midwives who were.

*When we women are not the centre of our care, **reality** is define, not by us, the birthing woman, but by the (often absent) doctor. And so in my cameo, what carried weight was not my description of what was happening to me, nor the opinion of a trained midwife's examination, but only the hands of the doctor. Only she or he could inform me that I was in second stage.*

One of the most shocking things I find about the medical literature is how little medicine thinks to ask the woman! And so we have a culture of disbelief which does not consider or validate women's experience of birth. It is, of course, only the doctor who knows what is going on… And so women have stopped believing in their bodies – they can no longer read its messages, and midwives are trained to defer to doctors and machines rather than their own eyes and hands and expertise of physiological birth.

*It is a phenomenon that has its roots in women's socio-cultural standing through history. The feminism of the sixties did not challenge it, **but we must** in order to retain, indeed reclaim, our dignity as birthing women, mothers and midwives.*

Furthermore, the historical dominance of the male doctor and the medicalisation of birth has produced a false dichotomy between the welfare of the mother and that of the baby, pitting the welfare of one against that of the other. The most common example is to tell the mother that she is putting the baby AT RISK if she does not do as she is told. I have mercifully been spared this experience but so many friends and customers have been threatened with the dreadful risks to their baby of having a home birth – sometimes even after the healthy baby has been born!

But more insidiously, the medical orthodoxy tells women unhappy with their treatment at birth, that they should stop complaining and be grateful for the healthy baby received from their hands. It took me to my fourth child to make a complaint about the care at my birth. Their response was of this very kind – as if the birth of a healthy baby was down entirely to them and I did not play any major role.

*What I want to say LOUD AND CLEAR is that a healthy mother and baby do not excuse substandard care, lack of respect and unnecessary intervention. We women want it all – a healthy baby **and** a positive birth, and we are entitled to expect BOTH without apology or qualification. What makes a good birth is not an ideal birth, but one where we are satisfied that what happened was as right as it could be and we had the support we needed. This false dichotomy is a product of our social standing as women, and the centrality of the medical perspective of birth.*

We need to challenge it.

And midwifery. *The midwives who had been so central to my care at home, who had been confident and competent professionals, became invisible under the bright hospital lights. I remember my GP, the late Dr Eisner, God bless her, confronting every doctor who walked into the room with the words, "I am Dr Eisner. Mrs Weston is my patient and she will want all the interventions explained and discussed with her." The midwives said nothing. Not out of a lack of compassion, but because they were not independent professionals in that setting, but simply servants, doing as they were told. And for me as the woman, that rendered me both vulnerable and alone because I had no advocate and no protection.*

The demise of the independent professional midwife has its roots in the socio-economic discrimination of women and midwives through the centuries, and has been documented by greater souls than mine such as Marjorie Tew[4], but I can offer you the contemporary results from a user's perspective:

The midwife in hospital (and increasingly in the home) has become silent and complicit in the mistreatment of birthing women and their partners. They act outside their own professional code, their human compassion and sometimes downright common sense and medical evidence, in order to fulfil their contract with the medical-led hierarchy, their Hospital Trust. Even independently-minded NHS midwives conspire with the system, becoming what my mentor John Vincent calls, "the soft underbelly of the oppressive state," mitigating the cruelty with kind words and ameliorating the rules with subversive practices. I don't denounce the care but we do need to recognise its limitations.

Please let me be clear. I am not denigrating NHS midwives as individuals; in fact, the courage of midwives who advocate for women from within the system cannot be underestimated and has my total respect. However, for women to get the care they need, we need everyone to be clear about the consequences of midwives complicity in, and enslavement to, the current medical system. By enslavement I mean that midwives often have no choice — they have no autonomy in their speech and action.

So, what are we going to do about it? How can we change the scenario and turn the young midwife of my story into a confident professional? How can I receive the care of a midwife whom I can trust not to leave me in the crisis, but who will be my advocate and support my birth and choices? How can I ensure my choices and decisions are respected, and that birth policies are woman-centred and evidence-based rather than medical custom and practice-based?

Making Change Happen:
Disrupting the Patterns

This book is about providing an understanding about why things are the way they are and why it is so difficult to change them, learning how to spot power and interest in the words and policies of decision-makers – and to be able to pinpoint or trace back to where it lies. And finally, to learn the ways that ordinary people can disrupt these patterns of power to give ourselves and others space to gain power and autonomy over our bodies and/or our midwifery profession.

I used to talk confidently about change-making and I have sung at many false dawns. Now, 30 years later, I think the patriarchal power within NHS maternity care may be too strong to overturn; I think we can only disrupt. Disruption is about interrupting the normal routine or pattern of how things are done to make room for someone or something different to occur. Even though the difference only affects some people, or only survives for a short while, or removes only one injustice, it is still worth doing because hundreds and indeed thousands can gain the birth or care they deserve, until that opportunity is shut down. And then we conspire to disrupt again to open another opportunity for change to occur. I want to hand down the tactics I have used effectively, and indeed still use, to disrupt the patterns of patriarchy and power within maternity care and beyond.

What is important to say at this point, is that although there is much tragedy here, there is also laughter. Disrupting the system can be fun – to a certain extent, it should be fun, playful even, witty. The playfulness, the humour, the twinkle in the eye, humanises the system that dehumanises maternity care and its staff; it pokes fun at pomposity and challenges authority to not take itself so seriously. It is Holy Mischief, playing the Fool in the Shakespearean sense, it is a wake-up call to healthcare workers to come to their senses and return to their true vocation.

A Short Tutorial on Resistance

In that speech back in 2003, I gave a short and succinct lesson in the different forms of resistance. I share that lesson now, slightly altered and amended for its purpose here.

There are three ways to work against an oppressive system:

- Subversion

- Avoidance

- Confrontation

Subversion

Subversion, I suggest, is what many midwives and mothers practise now. Here are a couple of personal examples: After my second miscarriage, when I refused my D&C[5], I was put under enormous pressure by doctors. In between one of the rounds, I sat on a stool in the laundry room and sobbed – because, after all, I was a grieving mother – and a nurse came in and put her arms around me and whispered in my ear, "It's your body, love; you do what you want with it."

She was practising subversion, as was the midwife at one of my births who said, "I should call the ambulance and have you transferred right now but I am not going to. You are going to have your home birth."

Mothers subvert the system, often unconsciously, by smiling sweetly, doing their own thing and then calling the midwife too late to be able to do anything about it. As you will learn in Part 1, we used this tactic often: for instance, to avoid speaking to my consultant at my first birth, or to ensure I had a water birth with my fourth birth.

Subversion is the valid defiance of the powerless and I want to encourage it. Like rabbit burrows and woodworm, subversion can undermine big structures and edifices. But I doubt whether it will be enough to bring the whole system tumbling down, even if it grinds it to a halt. We need to do **more**.

Avoidance

Avoidance is another form of opposition. It is practiced by parents and midwives alike, where you circumvent or bypass the system altogether. You become an independent midwife or you engage an independent midwife, or go to a birthing centre, or even plan a freebirth (birth without a midwife or other qualified person). Some mothers have even left the country in search of the birth they want.

This action is costly for the protagonists. Midwives give up security and income and invite the hostile attentions of the medical establishment. The families who engage independent midwives or birthing centres pay substantial sums – for us fifth time around, it represented nearly 20% of our then income. Freebirth invites the hostile attentions of the medical establishment – for how is a mother to give birth without a medic to ensure she does it correctly?!

Those of us who have practised avoidance one way or another and have paid handsomely for the privilege will probably say that one way or another, it is worth every penny and every sacrifice. Whilst it can be a difficult road, we must recognise it is an important part of the opposition because it is providing an alternative model and practice. It demonstrates the alternative as realistic, workable and effective. Like the radicals and nonconformists of the past, we must take courage and be proud. We have done it because, to reclaim a commercial slogan, "We are worth it."

Confrontation

Confrontation. Ah, this is the difficult one because we are so well-conditioned not to make a fuss and to do as we are told. And, of course, we cannot win because if we are 'nice', nobody listens but if we get angry, we are dismissed as emotional, neurotic and stroppy women. Sadly, the feminism of the last century has not overturned these cultural norms, particularly in the maternity services. But I want to state clearly that silence is complicity and doing nothing for change is actively supporting the status quo. Ultimately, to bring about change, we **must** confront the beast and bring it down.

My husband, Dr David Weston, is an archaeologist and he says that ancient human hunters knew that they could not kill large prey like bison and mammoth with one shot of their little arrows. So they made arrows that did not kill but instead made very messy wounds. They aimed arrow after arrow at the beast, making such a bloody mess that the beast finally bled to death. We may not be strong enough to bring the beast down with one shot, but if we fire arrow after arrow at our prey, aiming to make as big a mess as we can with our puny arrows, it will finally fall bleeding from a thousand wounds. It is not a pleasant picture but it illustrates the tactic very well.

There is a problem with this tactic, in that as with me, women and parents find the moment of confrontation happens at our weakest point on enemy ground. And so I would say we need to organise; we do not simply need advice, we need advocacy. We need to demand implementation of professional standards that respect a woman/birthing person's decision. And we need someone at the consultation, in the meeting or at the birth acting as a witness, to support and advocate. For midwives, there is the bullying culture, the fear, the fragmentation, the lack of cohesion. Unfortunately, this is the norm for oppressed groups. It reminds me of some advice the late veteran MP Tony Banks once gave to a new MP: "Your opponents sit opposite you; your enemies sit behind you". I suspect that if you work for change, some of your toughest and most hurtful opposition will come from colleagues from within the NHS. Be prepared for that and start thinking of ways to deal with it.

Modelling the Alternative

The three forms of resistance are joined by a fourth: the positive modelling of alternatives. This can be seen in some of the acts of avoidance such as being or hiring an independent midwife, but it can also be seen as the work done to build alternative models of midwifery and maternity care WITHIN the system. We can only salute the leadership and sacrifices of many midwives who have advocated, set up and run home birth and/or case-loading teams, or midwifery-led birth units – fighting budget and staffing cuts for years to model this good practice. Caseloading at its simplest is where a midwife or small team takes on a reasonable caseload of women who they see throughout the maternal pathway – antenatal, birth and postnatal. This is often associated with the term 'Continuity of Midwifery Carer'.

We can only stand in awe of the midwives who have risked all, financially and professionally, to set up independent midwifery practices seeking to be commissioned into the NHS in the manner of GP practices (it could be an oversimplification but gives the picture). It is no fault of these midwifery-led practices that they failed, despite modelling excellence and with impressive outcomes. For the NHS system, mired in its historic gender inequality, power and control are more important than impressive rates of physiological birth and family satisfaction.

These examples show how modelling the alternative is tough, very tough in some cases. The reason it is so tough is because in a very positive and inspiring way, it resists the status quo; it disrupts the accepted order. Of course, the reflex of those made powerful in the current system is to be threatened by such positive modelling, because the impressive outcomes of, for instance, caseloading midwifery teams, holds their managers and commissioners accountable for their own dismal failure to deliver the same outcomes in their system. This is why, readers, the history of maternity in the UK is littered with closed birth centres, burnout caseloading teams and malicious referrals to the Nursing and Midwifery Council. Be in no doubt, seeking to set up and actually running positive alternative models, such as caseloading and midwifery-led units, is an effective act of resistance and will be viewed as such.

Changing the Way the Wind Blows

My experience of working with deprived groups in Britain is that what you need is a few motivated people getting together in a particular place at a particular time to change things which then impact more widely: the ripple effect. For instance, Airedale Mums got together at a particular time and place to make changes in THEIR hospital, but their impact was felt far wider.

Part 1 tells the story of my own wake-up call to act for change in maternity care. I reflect on the care I received and the key issues it raises for maternity services generally. The substance of the book, Part 2, is about getting together, organising and building allies, and running campaigns to effect change. I share the skills and tactics I have been taught and which we have used to good effect. It is about how to deal with difficult conflict situations when they come your way, as they inevitably will.

Part 3 is for anyone near burnout or ready to give up, and is where I share something of my story. However, in a practical way, I look at strategies for prevention and survival of burnout, reflect on the causes and conditions that break us and remake us, and recognise and endorse the importance of the different roles activists play when the front line is not for them. However, I must be clear, this is no Haynes Manual for activism, I do not cover every scenario! What I do is give you pointers, tips, tasters and warnings, to help you form your own action and spot 'red flags', so you are not completely surprised, ambushed or broken.

We need groups of parents and midwives to band together to write letters, set up petitions and plan protests to challenge current maternity policy, nursing and midwifery regulation, and change legislation. We need people who are witty, creative, techno-literate and media-savvy who band together to change the way the wind blows...

Because it is important to grasp, that politicians – at Westminster, the Town Hall, NHS Commissioners and managers – are wet fingered: they hold their wet fingers up to SEE WHICH WAY THE POLITICAL WIND IS BLOWING! (Jim Wallis)[6]

And so it is true to say that change will happen not so much by replacing one wet-fingered politician with another, but as much as changing the way the political wind blows. As ordinary women and men, we may not be able to change the actual people making the decisions, but we do have it within our power to change the way the political wind blows: that is the criteria, the culture, the context in which those decisions are made.

We need to be determined, clever, fun.

We need to band together to organise and unionise, to write letters and demonstrate.

And we need to educate, educate, educate.

Talk to our daughters, sisters, mothers;

Talk to our sons, husbands, brothers;

And we need to fearlessly claim our heritage to birth and bring to birth,

To be the women, the mothers, the midwives we are.

We need to campaign as determinedly and creatively as we give birth,

Because our daughters are worth it

— and so are we.

Part 1

~

Birth of an Activist

A Note for the Confused

When you have five births and two miscarriages in one book, it can get confusing! I don't use the medical jargon but I do follow their rule in that I count pregnancies separately to live births, so I have had seven pregnancies but only five live births. This means that when I talk about my first birth, second birth etc., I am NOT talking about the miscarriages but am only numbering my *living children and their births*. I will occasionally use my children's name in the text (they are really good names!) but generally speaking, I will talk about them in numbers because it makes it easier for readers to follow…!

Chapter 1

✧

The Wake-up Call

I CAME TO BIRTH ACTIVISM as a trained liberation theologian and as a community organiser and activist in Bradford. I grew up in a mining area during the miners' strike, and spent significant portions of my life living in deprived urban areas. In Bradford, I set up a national student poverty campaign through the church and chaplain network I was part of, and facilitated a student housing campaign that resulted in improvements in policy that are still in place today. I was involved in a number of local projects, from the Housing Action Group to a support group for a local ex-offenders' hostel. However, I did not apply my knowledge and skills to maternity at first because it was personal, and I thought I would not need to. How wrong I was!

The First Wake-up Call

The first wake-up call was 13 weeks into my first pregnancy when I was referred to hospital with a suspected miscarriage. It was 4th August 1993. My husband was not allowed to accompany me into the ultrasound scan and I was not allowed to see the screen. Nothing was explained to me. I was returned to the ward, and 30 minutes later a junior doctor arrived to read out the statement I had heard the sonographer type out in my presence but seemed unable to say: that there was no heartbeat, that the baby was dead. Of course, I did not understand the system or the technology and so I refused to believe it.

"Show me!" I demanded.

I was told that if I insisted, it could be arranged but would mean losing my place in the surgery queue and therefore an overnight stay. This is a ploy I came to recognise and learnt to subvert in future encounters. It was a God-awful place and I did not want to stay one moment longer than necessary and so I caved in – but there was that nagging doubt that tortured me for months afterwards. I was recommended a D&C, as was standard in the area, to remove the remains, and I accepted because I did not know any better.

The operation was not successful in any of the ways I was told it would be: it did not remove all the remains, it did not prevent pain, and it did not prevent a womb infection. I suffered enormously over many months and even years from this miscarriage, and perhaps it was at this point, rather than any other incident, where I lost my trust in the medical system to always tell me the truth and care for my needs.

The Moral of This Tale:

- Do not accept what you are told simply because you are told it by a clinician.

- You can do any or all of the following: Ask for the evidence base or guideline that this clinical opinion is based on. Ask for a second opinion. Ask for any statistic to be set out with a common denominator i.e. 1 in 10,000 chance, not just "higher risk".

- Ask questions and know that you have the right to take all the time you need to make the decision that is right for you.

- Ask for the care you need. Get your family to demand the care you need.

- You can leave hospital and go home to get some space if you want to, or simply go and spend some time off the ward.

- But also remember that in this situation we are vulnerable and sometimes we cannot assert ourselves and our needs. Do not be hard on yourself if you cannot assert your needs, because it is their job to be kind, not yours to be assertive.

- Finally, be kind to yourself and give yourself plenty of time to recover from your loss.

The Second Wake-up Call

The second wake-up call came in the next pregnancy, of child number one, my daughter Hannah. It was 1994. The policy of the time was that every woman during her pregnancy should have one consultation with the consultant assigned to them. I am not sure why a low-risk woman under midwifery care needed to have a named consultant nor why she needed to see him (and it was "him" in those days) – but there we are! At that time I did not know better, and, frankly, still grieving for the loss of Hilda (the name I gave to my miscarried baby) a few months before, I did not care. By the end of the consultation, however, I did care very much.

The consultation started off as expected. There were two midwives present; the doctor arrived and gave me a perfunctory examination on the bed. He then sat down at the desk, looking for all the world like a bank manager, sat proprietarily in suit and tie. Meanwhile, I sat mostly dressed on the edge of the bed, swinging my legs like a schoolgirl. He asked me if I had any questions. Well, actually I did. I had recently read an interesting account in a local newspaper about a woman having a water birth and what a difference it made to her. I thought I might like one too. His response took me aback.

"Do you mean to say, you want to endanger your baby's life by having it under water? Only whales and dolphins have babies under water!"

He then went on to tell me about a couple of incidents where a baby had died during a water birth. I was aware of these but puzzled because it was not the water birth as such that was the cause of death. However, I sat mute. I felt like a 10-year-old in front of an angry headmaster. He then told me that the unit was going to have a birthing pool installed possibly in time for my birth.

Clearly, he was concerned that women would birth in the pool against his wishes because he went on to say, "No woman of mine will refuse to get out of the pool when I tell her to."

He swept out of the room and I was left to finish dressing with two embarrassed midwives who said nothing: they were as mute and powerless as I was. The stroppy woman inside me, the inner feminist, silenced by grief for so long, spoke loud and clear in my head. I remember the words to this day: *If you don't take back control over your body now, that man will have all the say in what happens. No man is going to tell me what I can and cannot do with my own body!* I did not want him or his hands anywhere near me again. I did not know how I was going to do it, but no one, especially that man, was going to treat me like that again.

The first thing I decided to do was to change my consultant so I would not encounter him or his attitudes again. I contacted my GP, who delivered my maternity care alongside the nearby hospital, and told him that I wanted to change my consultant. I thought it a straightforward request but I had not encountered the power and hierarchy of the medical system. He did not say no, but he was clearly uncomfortable and embarrassed, and nothing was done.

What I did not know until later was that the consultant was a member of the hospital senate – a very powerful man in the local medical world. And I had just told my GP that I did not want anything more to do with him! We lived in a flat above the medical practice so we knew the staff.

The practice manager heard what had happened and drew me to one side one day. She handed me a piece of paper and said quietly to be out of earshot, "My daughter is a midwife. You need to talk to the midwives. Here is their phone number."

What a breath of fresh air! There, in a consulting room in Kensington Street Medical Centre, Ann Devanny opened up to me a world of possibilities that I did not know existed.

"You would not have to meet Mr C if you had your baby at home," was her take on my predicament.

"But I thought you could only have your second baby at home!" I gasped. I had read an account of a home birth years before and had thought then, *If ever I get to have a baby, that is the way I want to birth it.* And that was how I came to book my first home birth.

Of course, it was not as simple as that. In those days you had to have GP cover but only one GP in the whole of Bradford provided cover for home births… so at 38 weeks pregnant, not only did I book a home birth under midwifery care, but I had to change my GP to a practice two bus rides away. God bless, Ann Devanny and Dr Eisner!

A postscript to this tale is that once I had booked my home birth, I received a call from the consultant's PA. She said he wished me to make an appointment to discuss my decision with him. After the 'whales and dolphins' debacle, it was not a discussion I wanted to have, especially on his ground, but I did not feel I could say an outright no to this powerful personage. I had been warned this might happen and so I prepared a genius response – I don't know where it came from.

I said, "I would be happy to discuss my decision with Mr C; my door is always open, and so we could make an appointment for him to see me at my home?"

There was a pause, then the PA responded smoothly that she would pass the message on to Mr C and get back in touch. I heard nothing more.

The Moral of This Tale:

- ALWAYS remember: it is your body, your baby, your decision.

- Seek knowledgeable and experienced allies to help you skilfully navigate the maternity system.

- Seek support and advocacy to avoid seeing healthcare professionals (HCPs) who act with impunity and who do not uphold the values we expect – nor indeed the values of their professional codes of practice.

- Challenges and obstructions in your pregnancy can sometimes be the catalyst for positive change, where you empower yourself with information, seek out an ally or support group, or take an alternative path. As I said to my midwives before the birth, I ought to send a postcard of thanks to Mr C because if it had not been for him, I would

never have sought out the midwives and booked the home birth I really wanted!

- **This was an act of subversion. Use these methods to get what you want or avoid unwanted attention when you are not powerful enough to act directly.**

Hannah's birth did not go to plan. Babies never pay attention in antenatal classes.

I don't want to go into the details of the birth as it is not what the book is about, but I do want to highlight a couple of points. I spent 18 of the 24 hours I was birthing at home. There I found the midwives to be competent, skilled and kind. I was treated with respect, and more than that, I was treated as if I was someone truly special, the centre of their attention. They did everything in their power to keep my birth both physiological and at home. They were committed to enabling me to have a good birth and were genuinely sad that this would not happen. After the birth, they were solicitous of not only my physical health but also my mental health. They talked things through with me, encouraged me, believed in me: they set me back on my feet.

By contrast, when transferred into hospital for slow progress and possible meconium, the experience was totally different. I was not the centre of attention, I was not special and there was a profound lack of kindness that was both personal and systemic. The midwives who had been so central to my care at home, who had been confident and competent professionals, became invisible under the bright hospital lights.

I remember my GP, God bless her, confronting every doctor who walked into the room with the words, "I am Dr Eisner, Mrs Weston is my patient and she will want all the interventions explained and discussed with her."

The midwives said nothing. Not out of a lack of compassion but because they were not independent professionals – they were not my midwives, but the hospital's midwives. And for me as the woman, that rendered me both vulnerable and alone because I had no advocate and no protection. The hospital lights not only rendered the midwives invisible, but also unable to fulfil their professional role without supervision from a doctor.

Hours passed. I was in agony, my labour augmented by synthetic hormones, no pain relief. My GP had to leave to start her clinic. The midwives left to care for other women. Suddenly in the madness of pain, I felt a change, a chink of light in my soul, I felt something had shifted.

My companions buzzed for the midwife. A midwife we had not seen before appeared and, after an examination, said, "You are 10 cm but let a doctor check you."

I was genuinely puzzled. "Why? Where is the doctor?" I asked.

"Doctor will be here in about 15 minutes," came the reply.

"I have been labouring for 24 hours! I am NOT waiting for any doctor! You are a midwife – do your job!"

Never in a month of Sundays would my community midwives have considered summoning a doctor to check if I was fully dilated!

When it came to the actual birth, I gave birth in agony facing a blank wall and a drip machine, because no one thought me important enough to speak to my face – they simply shouted instructions from my rear. When I shouted, 'I cannot hear you – come and speak to my face!!' they ignored me and just shouted louder. I call this birth my crucifixion. Kindness would have mitigated that agony – but there was no kindness.

Where was the kindness? I was doing an amazing and courageous thing birthing my baby, and the more difficult the birth, the greater the courage required. After the birth, a midwife (I think) took me to have a bath. As I tottered down the corridor behind her, she explained that she was very busy with a delivery of supplies so I could only have 10 minutes. She put me in the bath and left me. Alone for the first time, I cried and cried. I have no words for the feelings of that moment but I would not want any of my children to be in that place without comfort. When the midwife returned, she told me off for not soaping myself down, so I dried my tears and did as I was told. I was a grown woman, for goodness sake! I had just given birth after 24 hours of labour and an augmentation! Where is the kindness? Where is the respect?

By contrast: at home, at my second birth (my eldest son), my community midwife Madge plonked herself right in front of me, face to face and said, "We are going to do this – woman to woman!"

And we did.

After the birth, Madge and her team wrapped me in towels and a dressing gown and helped me from the bed to the warm bath they had run for me. I was attended by a friend and my daughter whilst they cleaned up and made my bed. Then they came into the bathroom with towels, helped me out of the bath, dried me, dressed me, put me into bed and placed the child in my arms. I felt like a queen. I was full to overflowing with love and happiness. The midwives told me afterwards that they were distressed to hear me asking over and over again, "Why are you doing this? Why are you doing this? I did not have this last time. I did not have this last time!" which was when I needed it more.

Their response was, "It's our job, this is what we do!"

For these community midwives, kindness was their job. And kindness makes all the difference.

Back in hospital with baby number 1 (Hannah), I was now on the postnatal ward and attempting that all-important first wee. I was not told how painful it could be! I cried out.

Thinking something was wrong, I pulled the cord; a smart young midwife came to the door. With tears in my eyes, I said that weeing really hurt. She looked at me like I was something on the bottom of her shoe and said, "Use the bidet," and walked off! I was a working-class girl and had no idea what a bidet was! So I tottered along the corridor and found the bathroom. The bath was dirty, so I cleaned it – although my head and legs felt like they were held together by a length of fraying string – ran the bath, got in and had a wee in relative comfort. Where is the kindness? I had cleaned a bath after 24 hours of labour but was not allowed to carry my own baby out of the ward? What kind of care is that?

The Wake-up Call:
What I learned

If I thought this first birth was 'just my bad luck', that it was 'one bad apple', one bad experience, then I would not be writing a book. It is not just my bad luck, nor one bad apple; this lack of human kindness is systemic. Systemic means that a lack of human kindness is built into the system – it means that no matter how kind you are as a person and as a health professional, the system forces you to behave in ways that are ultimately unkind towards the women and people you should be caring for.

And because of the historic place of women in our society and culture, we as women – midwife and mother – submit to it, assume it is the norm and therefore okay. But it is NOT okay and NEVER has been. It was only the contrast in care between home and hospital that alerted me to the fact there was something wrong. It was only reading an article about PTSD in a birth activist magazine[7] a few years later that told me that my flashbacks and trauma were normal responses to the experience I had suffered – something the maternity system still barely acknowledges, let alone takes responsibility for.

In the intervening years, I have read and listened to countless of birth stories that echo my story – the details change but the common themes of hard medical intervention, coercion, feeling vulnerable and unprotected, lack of kindness, lack of respect, not being listened to. Thirty years of suffering and the maternity system is still is not effectively held to account, and is still not listening to what women are saying.

What I have learnt in my years of activism is that in this great country of ours, in our fabulous NHS, we have taken the care out of maternity and created a factory system which puts little value on kindness and humanity. Midwives and indeed clinicians are not paid to be skilled and kind; they are paid to ensure throughput, to ensure good outcomes. The good outcomes being a living mother and baby discharged home. Frankly, I feel that getting out alive is a very low bar for care!

Mental and emotional well-being is not important; being listened to, respected and supported is not in the package – they are add-ons in the system, 'nice to haves' which good midwives and clinicians make every effort to deliver, **but**, and this is significant, it is ON TOP OF THEIR WORK, rather than integral to it[8].

As one senior midwife remarked to me a few years later, "Unfortunately, there is no measure for TLC and so our work is not measured on how kind we are."

My view is that the maternity system is structurally misogynistic because it puts the well-being and smooth running of the system over and above the well-being and needs of the women and their families that pass through. Women get the feeling that they are rather an inconvenience to the smooth running of maternity services, and indeed they are. The system is truly misogynistic because it not only crushes the woman, but it crushes the midwife: historically, the maternity system with its patriarchal hierarchy was designed to sideline and silence midwives too.

Chapter 2

~

Doing It My Way

Doing It *My* Way:
The Second Miscarriage

I FOUND AND PAID FOR some good therapy in the coming years and the next two pregnancies healed the previous two.

In 1996 I fell pregnant again, unexpectedly. But at eight weeks pregnant, on 4th August – the exact same date of my previous miscarriage – I had the same show that indicated the termination of the pregnancy. I was staying with my parents and so I rang their GP, a lovely Irishman, who told me there was probably little to be done and he did not want to send me off to hospital. He suggested I continued the stay with my parents with bed rest, and contact my GP when I returned home. I had two gentle days, nurtured by family, to come to terms with my loss and prepare for what might happen next.

I returned home and rang the GP and my therapist. This time I was going to do things differently, but I was going to need help and support. I told my GP that I did not want to go to the hospital if I was treated the way I was last time. She therefore wrote a letter which I took with me stating that not only was I to be treated with care, but that I should be able to see the scan and have everything explained to me.

Then it came to the discussion of what to do about the miscarriage. The junior doctor, four days into her rotation, gave me the same 'talk' as last time about how a D&C to remove the remains was safer, preventing pain and bleeding. I told her the story of my last miscarriage, commenting that the benefits were not the experience of myself or any friend I had spoken to who had had one. She had little to say in response, maybe because she knew less than I did. Without a compelling reason for a D&C, I was minded to refuse, but I was unwilling to do so in my vulnerable state on someone else's home ground, so I took the tactic of avoidance. I said that I had received some very sad news and I did not want to be rushed into any decision, so I wanted to go home and spend time with my family coming to terms with our loss, and we would get back to them in the morning. The doctor was clearly trying to be empathetic; nonetheless, like last time, I was warned of the possible dire consequences of going home. But this time, I was adamant. We left the hospital, collected my daughter from nursery and we spent a happy couple of hours mucking about on the allotment – it is a memory full of joy even now.

I rang my therapist; she said she would support me if I chose to have a natural miscarriage. She talked me through it and said I needed to ring her daily. She would provide remedies to help. I rang my GP.

"I don't want a D&C."

She mused about how different people are. In her family, they had moved heaven and earth – or at least districts – to enable her sister-in-law to have a D&C following a miscarriage.

Then she said, "You are not like other women so I will tell you the truth."

And the truth of the matter was that the risk that worried everyone was haemorrhage, and according to the data, the risk was slightly greater if you had a miscarriage naturally.

"How much greater?"

She stopped my questions gently.

"Ruth, this is not about what the research says, this is about you and your decision."

And I realised it was. I had made my decision and I was simply looking for justifications. Then she told me she would support me in my decision to have the miscarriage naturally as long as I rang her every two or three days to give her an update. Truly another doctor who hides wings and a crown! Here was a healthcare worker who provided me with unbiased information, helped me acknowledge the decision I had already made and then supported me – even though it was clear it was not a decision she would have made for herself or her loved ones.

It took two weeks to miscarry. I had a normal labour with contractions. Perhaps I am the only woman in the world who invited someone to sell me a kitchen whilst labouring a miscarriage! I have to say, it was a fun and effective distraction and I would recommend it – it was an unbelievable story for the woman to tell her colleagues the next morning too. I never managed to thank her properly.

It was a good labour and birth; but without an experienced 'midwife', I panicked at the end and we called an ambulance. This was a big mistake and it cost me dear: I was deprived of the love and company of my husband through that long night; the remains were taken away and despite my request to have them returned for burial, they were not; and I was back in the medical system I had wanted to avoid with all its cruelties. I faced the registrar alone to refuse the D&C again, having had 12 hours nil by mouth. I escaped with some heavy-duty antibiotics as a preventative of infection – the irony that my womb infection came from the D&C was absolutely clear but I saw it as a straight bargain for my freedom.

One further point: the nurses had told me I could discharge myself. They also told me that if I did not intend to have the operation, I might as well eat. But refusing medical advice when you know so little is really scary, and without support there with me, I could not do it alone.

Part of the bargain for my freedom was the commitment to return in a week's time to check there were no 'retained products'. Unfortunately, the next week, the scan did show some retained products and so the pressure to have the D&C resumed. I refused. Why were they so concerned about retained products after a natural miscarriage and totally oblivious to retained products from their D&C? I was causing trouble and so the junior doctors passed me between themselves before passing me up the pole to their superiors. I refused to go back into the public waiting room in my distressed state, and so between rounds I ended up sitting on a stool in the laundry room, crying my eyes out, because after all I was a bereaved mother – something that seemed to be forgotten!

As I sat sobbing alone, a nurse came into the room, hugged me close to her and whispered fiercely in my ear, "It's your body, love; you do what you want with it."

She left my side before I could see who she was – another angel I cannot thank.

I do remember later being moved into an office with the junior doctors who I had met earlier. I think we were all waiting for the judgement from on high because we chatted as equals and not as opponents. I remember asking where their research and data came from for the advice they gave. "From the medical text book," came the answer.

"So where and when did that data come from?" I wondered. I was taken aback that they did not know the evidence on which their advice was based. I commented tactfully that I would want the references to check them out.

For their part, they asked me about what it was like to have a natural miscarriage. I remember the astonishment of one of the doctors (both were female) when I told her that for pain and general well-being, I would have a 10-hour labour and birth any day of the week rather than a D&C. "It was right and beautiful," I told her. My comments landed with her, and hopefully she is a better doctor for it.

The judgement from on high came at last: I was free to go. They would not try to coerce me anymore. So I left hospital, returned home, and cried and cried and cried, all my courage and fortitude spent.

The Moral of This Tale:

- Within the medical system, you can make real choices, but it takes an enormous amount of courage to act against 'medical advice', or what is in reality 'medical coercion'.

- You can find professionals who will tell you the truth and support your decision-making with perception and tenderness. They are more precious than gold.

- Luck plays a big part in what happens – but so do you. Your wisdom and courage bear fruit.

- There are kind people working in the hospital who will subvert the system to support you.

- Often your opponents, the doctors, are good people trying to do their job well and according to what they have been taught. But remember that what they have been taught is not always right for you.

- When unkindness is systemic, it does not matter how nice people are; the system makes them say and do cruel things. When the system is more important than the people it purports to serve, then it should be dismantled, because it can do

as much harm as good. Doctors make an oath about that.

Doing It *My* Way:
The Birth of My Second Child

It is now 1998: my fourth pregnancy and the birth of my second child. I had learnt from my first miscarriage so left a gap between miscarriage and another pregnancy, falling pregnant the first cycle after the first anniversary of my loss. I researched optimal foetal positioning and spent *a lot* of time leaning forward to make sure that baby was in the best position for an easy birth. I also hired a birthing pool. We still had no money but if this was to be my last child and after the suffering of the previous birth, I wanted anything that would make things easier.

Although Mr C was not my consultant this time, it was clear that the 'whales and dolphins' policy was still in force. And so it was, that although no consultant would grace my home birth, a midwifery manager was despatched to my home to inform me that it was not the policy to allow mothers to have water births as they were thought to be dangerous for "Ohhhh, lots of reasons!" and that if I still chose to do so, then on my head be it. We both signed to say we had discussed the issues, and that was that!

But the consultant still had to have his say in my birth, and so at 8 cm dilated, whilst I was in that tricky stage of transition, one of the midwives spoke up and said, "At this moment, I have to ask you to leave the pool as it is not Bradford Trust's policy to allow you to remain in the pool for the birth."

I politely refused and with that formality over with, we all prepared for my birth in water. What was absolutely clear from this farce was that although the consultant was not present at my physiological, low-risk, midwifery-led home birth on a Sunday afternoon, he was present in the actions and words of the midwives who were. Neither they, nor I, were autonomous even in my home.

This meant that because water birth was against hospital policy, it refused to furnish midwives with the appropriate equipment because that would tacitly accept women might birth in water. So, whilst I was deep into labour, a midwife asked, "We need a hand mirror. Have you got a hand mirror?"

We had, but my husband did not know where it was. I did. I was furious because every word required enormous and painful effort.

"There is a pile of five Bibles – Bible, Bible, Bible, Bible, Bible! On top of the five Bibles, there is the mirror!"

Madge, my woman-to-woman midwife, laughed and exclaimed, "Where is your sense of humour? Laughter gets the baby out!"

Grrr! The cheek of it!

I had my baby at home. I danced through this birth, swinging my hips to Duke Ellington, Fats Waller and The Big Band Swing! I birthed in the pool cheered on by my husband, my homeopath and five midwives! For community midwives, apparently my home water birth was a rare and wonderful thing and an opportunity for training. I was surrounded by love, held in kindness, and the room was filled with laughter and joy. I call this birth 'my ordination' because I felt I was co-creator with God in bringing this baby into the world, I was one with the dance of creation, love and joy mixed together – and surely that made me a priest, whatever the churches' view of women's priesthood! This birth was my ordination to priesthood and nothing and no one could take that conviction away from me. No one ever has.

My daughter was eating pasta when I birthed but half an hour later, she came to inspect Mum's empty tummy and view her baby brother, whom she immediately claimed as hers. My neighbour secretly put a sign in our window proclaiming, 'It's a boy!'

The Moral of This Tale:

- **Giving birth can and should be a joyous occasion full of love and laughter.**

- **The pain is real but with joy and love, it is overcome.**

- **Kindness has a real impact on the experience of pain. It can be a most effective pain relief and preventative of trauma.**

- **A good birth empowers a mother, and its good effects can change her forever.**

- **In this space, midwifery is the most wonderful profession. In this space, midwives fulfil their true vocation. And it is a travesty of love and life that this beautiful experience is denied so many** women and so many midwives because of an inhumane system that does not accept its own research and data.

- Obstetricians overstep the mark when they interfere in the normal physiological births and choices of women at home. Their specialism is pathologies of birth.

Doing It *My* Way:
My Millennium Baby (and Third Child)

The year 2000; I was never going to be so kitsch as to have a millennium baby – but I did! On the last day of March early one morning, I started in labour. Midwifery care in Bradford was fragmenting and so I could not be sure who would turn up for my birth. We were heartily relieved when Madge rang up to tell us she was on duty.

"I was praying it would be me!" she said.

There is nothing like that to make you feel special. The pain was sharp at the beginning and I was SOOO angry! But a remedy from the homeopath and I shifted a gear.

A few minutes later, I was in the pool swinging my hips and singing along to Fats Waller. We sang this baby out – five midwives, a homeopath, my husband and the wonderful Granny Jeanie, my friend, whose hands could rub a back like no other. I was worried that the contractions did not hurt enough – the midwives reassured me all was well.

I call this my Sacred Birth, because at a certain moment I felt like I was walking up the centre aisle of St David's Cathedral. When I reached the altar, my baby would be born.

However, the vision faded because fear crept in: the painful memories of this last bit scared me. I was scared of the pain. After a while, I turned to Madge and said, "I could have had the baby half an hour ago, but I don't like this last bit."

Madge gave me a pep talk, whilst the homeopath popped a remedy into my mouth and Jeanie began to say the St Patrick's Prayer of Protection I had pinned on the wall by the pool. Two contractions and one roar later, Tilly was born. All was confusion and noise. I wanted to lift the baby from the pool myself and someone else had done it and I was shouting for my baby, the baby was crying, everyone was talking and exclaiming and crying at once! That said, the photos Jeanie took of the birth are sensational and should be shared with the world one day.

This is still my favourite birth. Not because everything was perfect, or everything was done the way it should – I am sure my membranes were artificially ruptured without my consent and I had wanted to lift my baby from the water myself – but because it was full of friendship and joy, and singing and laughter. The birth was also short and relatively easy. Truly it was a Eucharist – a celebration!

This is a birth I would wish on all my friends and daughters, and on every midwife and doula. It does not have to be discussed; it just needs to be experienced and treasured. This sort of birth should be the bread and butter of midwifery, not a rare gem plucked from the grinding of the maternity machine.

The joy and the bath of birth hormones carried me along for some time. However, the challenge of this baby was caring for three young children on my own whilst my husband worked away. I teetered on the edge of postnatal depression – not because I had a bad birth, but because I lacked the practical support I needed to sustain the 24/7 shift that is parenthood. Maternity care in the UK stops far too early; a live mother and baby is not enough; we need to be healthy and happy as well.

Chapter 3

~⟡~

The Game Changer

The Third and Final Wake-up Call (Fourth Child)

THE YEAR WAS 2002. It was eight weeks before the birth of my fourth child. I rang to book the hire of my birthing pool from the Leeds-based midwife who had started Aquabirths.

"I am sorry, I can't. I will be in New Zealand in three weeks' time."

"Is this for a holiday?" I asked slowly.

"No, I am emigrating. Leaving in three weeks."

"So what will happen to the pools?"

"I'm selling the pools and the business."

"Can I hire a pool off the person buying it?"

"No one is buying the business."

"Oh… [long pause] So what will happen to the pools?"

"At this point? I will just leave them in the garage."

"Oh." [Another long pause]

And the community activist in me thought: If she leaves the pools in the garage, not only will I be unable to have a water birth, but neither will women all over Yorkshire – except at London prices shipped up here! We would not want that. We could not afford it.

"I'll take it on."

Just like that. The words came out of my mouth bypassing my rational brain.

"Really?"

"Yes. [Pause]… but oh! I should ask my husband!"

I rang my husband at work.

"Are you sat down? I have something I need to tell you."

"The washing machine has broken?"

"No. No. It's not that. I've bought a business. I have just bought the pool hire company – that's okay, isn't it?!"

"Oh. Yes, that's fine."

I could not quite believe it. He answered me in the same tone as if I had rung him to tell him the kettle had broken and I had just bought a new one! As if buying a business was just another 'fun thing' his batty wife might get up to whilst he was at work!

My parents turned up an hour later, popping in on their way home from somewhere. I told them what I had done. I was surprised by how pleased they were! This was good because I was a community organiser and I could set up projects and campaigns, but I had never set up or run a business before. Clearly, my parents thought I could do it.

This was Friday. On the following Tuesday, on my train to work, we agreed terms. On the Thursday, after work and the kids' teatime, we went over to her house where we were given paperwork and viewed the pools in the garage by torchlight. It was then we learnt she had booked an earlier flight and she was leaving on Sunday for her new life.

That was it. On Sunday 5th July 2002, we became the proud owners of Aquabirths Birthing Pool Hire. It was eight weeks before the birth of my fourth child and we had never run a business before. A few months later, my husband, myself and our baby son enrolled on a basic business course and so the adventure began!

It was the game-changer. The third and final wake-up call, when my work life/sense of vocation collided with, and became one with, my role as a mother. The personal became political. And I also meant business because it was my living. This was the moment when I threw in the towel and said, "Okay, I will do it! I will become a birth activist rather than a generic community organiser. Change-making not in the church or the community, but in maternity. Watch out! A force of nature has just been unleashed!"

The Birth of My Fourth Child

With the enormous amount of effort I put into obtaining a pool for my birth, one would have hoped that I could have birthed in it – but that was not to be.

The pool was set up and ready to go as labour cracked on. However, community midwifery had deteriorated in the eight years I had been having babies and, rather than a midwife I knew and trusted being there, attendance could be by any one of 70 odd midwives. I was consoled by the belief that an agreement was in place that the second midwife would be trained in water birth and I knew all of them: in fact, I had 'trained' some of them!

On the day, a stranger turned up in my home. She was pleasant but had never seen or done a water birth…! I said (or I waved at my supporters to say it as I was almost beyond words) this was okay as backup had been arranged for her. She rang her managers for the promised backup: it had not been arranged. There was that tense pause as the implications sunk in.

Then my husband, God bless him forever, piped up and said, "This is my third water birth, and Jeanie here has attended two. If Ruth wants to get in the pool, we know what to do, we will help."

Within 30 minutes, two water birth midwives were at our door, pulled out of clinics to attend this 'emergency' water birth. They were in the birth room trying to sort out what was what and who had the oxygen, etc.: no one had brought any because they had been pulled out of other tasks and everyone thought someone else would have some. It was disturbing me, so my husband and Jeanie sent them into another room to get themselves sorted out.

For me, this birth was deeply unsatisfactory. Internationally renowned obstetrician Michel Odent says regularly at his doula training sessions that for an easy birth, there needs to be quiet, privacy and darkness.[9]

I had chosen a room for its size and being sunny, but it was too bright and there were no curtains. There were lots of people coming in and out and talking, and lots of strangers, so there was a lack of privacy and quiet. My labouring was fast and furious, with contractions running together which I found difficult to sustain. It took all my effort to keep my focus and stay above the powerful contractions – the 'foetus ejection reflex', as Odent would call it: the ancient animal instinct that says, *This place is unsafe; have the baby quick and run to safety.* My waters broke into the pool and contained sludgy meconium, a sign of distress in the baby. This was no surprise to me, for it was a fast and furious birth! The midwives went into professional panic mode.

My wonderful midwife for birth number one (Hannah) had taken charge now. "You will have your baby at home but we will have to transfer the baby and you to hospital straight after."

"Okay."

"We need that baby out fast."

"This contraction or next?"

"My God, Ruth, give us time to get set up!"

I got out of the pool to birth the baby, and as I did so, the midwives were ringing for emergency ambulances. I felt very strong and, in a deep wordless place, I knew all was well – but my innate wisdom said I needed to stay focused and positive because if I panicked, then things would be really unsafe for the baby. So I said to my companions I must only hear positive words. And so the scene was set for a farcical cacophony as my husband and supporters shouted positive encouragement to drown out the voices of the midwives speaking to ambulance, clinicians, etc. preparing for an emergency. Of course, the midwives could not then be heard so they raised their voices, and so I birthed to a war of sound!

I birthed standing, quickly and painlessly. Standing to give birth was a lesson learnt for baby number 5 – it was sooooo easy compared with all fours or anything else! I would need a wheelie bin next time for the water birth! The benefits and safety mechanisms (all evidence-based) of intact cord and my own wishes were ignored for protocol[10]. The cord was cut immediately, the placenta blood (i.e. the baby's blood) bled out on the carpet. The baby was suctioned and then finally handed back to me.

I birthed the placenta but, of course, all the mechanisms were awry – and maybe in that cord cutting and removing of the placenta, the cord was tugged. A piece of placenta was left inside. The bleeding did not stop; there were some big clots. It was not gushing and scary, but not slow enough for the midwives to be happy. So off to hospital I went. The midwives and ambulance were kind, they did not rush me. The ambulance waited outside patiently whilst we enjoyed the triumph of birth. But then in we went.

The hospital was all fear and panic and worry, as a midwife every so often came in, examined the blood loss, grimaced, refused to give me any assurances, and left. I was terrified. After some hours, I persuaded a kind person to fill the wee pot with hot water, as I knew a trick from my days as a care assistant for releasing tissues. The warm steam relaxed my pelvic floor and a couple of litres of wee poured out and a lump of placenta popped out too. It seems that in our ultra-medical settings, we have lost the simple non-medical tricks of the trade.

When I was finally let out, I apparently had had a PPH (postpartum haemorrhage) because I had lost over 500 millilitres (estimated) of blood, but my blood count was something like 125 and I was fine. Was it a PPH? That is a whole other story and book, but for the purposes of this book, the key factor was that my husband and I were told that I had a PPH, that it happened in women and birthing people who had lots of babies, and that the risk increased the more babies you had.

The information was so out of date, it was a travesty of the phrase 'evidence-based medicine'.[11] But we did not know this until much later. A tangible result of this misinformation was that my husband did not sleep for weeks before the birth of my fifth child because he was afraid I might die and it would be his fault. Thank God for Michelle, our independent midwife, and her truly evidence-based approach to birth.

I returned home with baby number 4, both of us exhausted and hungry, to pick up the pieces and try to recover alongside our three other children. My husband had a week's 'compassionate' leave from work. Four weeks later, he was working away, then eight weeks later, he and I **both** had postnatal depression – yes, men get it too. The joy of childbearing and nursing were crushed by the lack of practical support again.

If we were the only family that faced this reality, I would not bother writing about it, but years of supporting families has taught me this is not the case. There seems to be a societal attitude that once the baby is born and you are home from hospital, you can just get on with it. There is a striking lack of understanding of the amount of physical and emotional work a small baby represents. It takes a tribe to raise a family and we leave it to two worn-out parents, one of whom has to go out to work 40 plus hours a week, leaving the other parent to fend for themselves.

By the end of the year and after being prescribed leave by his GP for work-related stress, my husband had changed roles in his firm to a lower paid one that kept him at home, and we set about looking for a more child-friendly career.

Chapter 4

✤

Building My Vision for Birth and Finding Independent Midwifery

MEANWHILE, AS WE recovered, I set about building Aquabirths into the vision I had of liberty for birthing women. Things moved fast.

The Letter of Complaint

I decided that I had had enough of putting up with whatever care was meted out to me and decided to finally make a formal complaint about the maternity care I received. I was drilled by the late Beverley Beech of AIMS (Chair of the Association for Improvements in the Maternity Services), so a letter was sent to everyone from the CEO of the Trust, supervisory regional people, the Chair of Parliamentary committees and the Health Secretary, as well as to my MP. It was early days for me in maternity activism so I could not read all the coded responses I received, which is a shame. However, the Trust's response was not coded: *I was only complaining out of commercial interest; and why was I complaining anyway? My baby and I were alive and well, what was there to complain about?*

How **dare** they?! I was furious and I dashed off a letter to my MP (he did not use email in 2003!). I expected him to contact the Trust, but not to forward my private angry letter to him with a note saying, "Sort this". The response of the Trust was a four-page apology... addressed to my MP, not to me. They forwarded him (not me!) the water birth policy with supporting references.

My husband read it aghast.

"If I used this level of evidence in my PhD, I would have failed it!"

Six thousand women a year were being treated under a guideline that deliberately lacked medical evidence. We Googled the references which were mainly from a neutral to positive Cochrane review (since updated).[12]

As the basis for denying every woman in Bradford a water birth for many years, the guidelines had picked out one negative piece of research which Cochrane noted was small scale, poor and lacked context. They also quoted a sentence from the whole document out of context and in so doing changed a positive reference into a negative one. We were appalled: we wrote a detailed critique of the policy, referencing it with prospective large-scale studies by respected European researchers that supported the safety of water birth (as opposed to the small scale one they used). The response? A short note saying they would not discuss the guideline with us. So this, my friends, was the state of medical guidelines in the UK in 2003. It was not scientific, not transparent; it was partial and based on the prejudices of the powerful in the service; it was not even open to challenge or accountability, even by those who suffered because of it. I wonder how far things might have improved in succeeding years?

I tried repeatedly to challenge Bradford Trust on the transparency and accountability of the guidelines. Even, a few years later, as Chair of the MSLC, with national guidelines to back me up, the clinicians were forceful and adamant that they would not share ANY guidelines unless a specific service user asked for a specific guideline, making transparency and accountability for service users impossible.

Meanwhile, my 2003 complaint and personal campaign ran into the sand because my then MP did not believe this sort of exchange of letters would get anywhere (he was probably right in a way) and withdrew his support for it. I would have to find another route to justice.

The First Choices in Childbirth Group

I set up a home birth group within months of baby no. 4 being born. It quickly changed its name to 'Choices in Childbirth' because as the group developed, it became clear that there were many choices parents needed to make, and place of birth was only one of them.

I was directed to the Yorkshire Storks Independent Midwifery Practice to support the group, because sadly NHS midwives are run off their feet and so do not have the supported time to facilitate empowering groups such as this. It was my first contact with independent midwives (IMs) and I was impressed. One Yorkshire Stork Midwife, Michelle Irving, knew answers to questions I did not know could be asked! She was self-deprecatory about her profession and practice; she could reference everything she told us. And she talked with respect, a light touch and lots of humour. Couples would turn up and go home open-mouthed with comments like, *"I never knew I could do that!"* and *"They [the healthcare professionals] never told me this!"* I soaked up the information like a sponge. But I learnt more than that: I learnt that my experiences of care were not unique; indeed, they were common practice. We learnt from parents about the latest local ruses for preventing women having home or water births, and provided our attendees with information and empowering techniques to get what they wanted.

To remind people of the date of the next meeting and to build attendance, I collected the email addresses of those who attended or were interested. Every month I would send out a quick email reminder. I then started adding in useful information, references shared at the meeting, and useful contacts and events coming up. The email grew longer and longer and so did the address list until the software crashed! And so it was the Choices e-newsletter was born, outgrowing the Choices group to become a thing in itself going out to doulas, midwives, mothers, heads of service and national organisations. It still does. The campaigning passion for empowerment, information and accountability shine through. You can still sign up to receive Choices.[13]

However, this was not enough for me. I became restless. Women were vulnerable to bullying, coercion and lack of or impartial information, and I wanted to tackle these issues at source, strategic level, with the Trust. But I was never invited to consultations, patient groups or anything like that. If I was invited to the big consultation day run by ASQUAM (Achieving Sustainable Quality in Maternity Services) every two years, then there would be nothing – even though I put my name down to be contacted again. Was I blacklisted? Or was it simply that they did not consult with women whoever they were? In the end, I started going to the Trust's AGM each year and asking questions there: they could not exclude me from that.

Growing Business and Family

As a Mum without a budget or time, I decided my marketing and campaign strategy was to raise my personal profile and talk to anyone and everyone about birth any time I had the opportunity. One definite target was to ensure that I was featured in the local newspaper one way or another every eight weeks, and I was! I have wonderful photos of me and the children in a birth pool together talking about liking it so much, I bought the company; of me and the children outside the house talking about tax credits; of me and the children outside our house holding home-grown veg talking about healthy eating; and so on and so forth.

It extended beyond the local paper, of course: our family were photographed for the NHS breastfeeding campaign with the quote: *"David's very good. He keeps the children occupied so I can just sit down and feed."* And somehow, I managed to persuade AIMS to let me give a 10-minute speech at the joint AIMS/ARM conference in Birmingham in spring 2003, with baby Stan who was just six months old. I received a standing ovation, much to my shock and surprise: I thought everyone said these things the way I did! The speech heads up the book, and its points have changed little in the last 20 years – which demonstrates the power of the patriarchal structures in UK maternity services.

Finally, encouraged by my business mentors to plan the expansion of our birth pool business from the start, I began setting up a nappy laundry service as a social enterprise – a project way before its time, aimed at reducing the carbon footprint and waste/pollution cycle of our babies. It absorbed an enormous amount of my time and energy, ultimately failing after three years when all we needed was £2,000 subsidy to cover the start-up costs for each new customer that joined us.

For the purposes of this story, the launch date of the service was to be autumn 2004… that is until I found myself pregnant with baby no. 5. I was devastated and embarrassed. But, as my dad said to me, "Well, you are good at having babies, so you might as well carry on!"

I dusted myself down and thought to myself, as I have no choice here I will have to use this pregnancy and birth to promote my passion for water birth, cloth nappies and good birth care – in any way possible. And that is how I ended up on the documentary series *Desperate Midwives*[14] as the woman that had a home water birth with an independent midwife.

Pregnancy and Birth With an Independent Midwife: The Difference

Michelle, the Choices midwife, now became Michelle **my** midwife, with her colleague Debs as my second midwife. She came an hour before the start of the monthly Choices group for my antenatals which were a revelation to me – less about the perfunctory physical checks, more about talking, learning, sharing information, building a relationship. Hopes and fears transpired and solutions were sought, plans were made and new information shared.

It was through such a conversation that my husband and I learnt that the information given to us about mothers being more likely to have a PPH the more children they have, was based on a survey done straight after the Second World War, when rationing was still in place! Imagine! The survey was repeated in the 1990s and showed this was no longer the case. Better nutrition had changed the outcomes.[15] It was a shame that the NHS had not updated its midwives because it caused an immense amount of unnecessary fear and suffering for me and especially my husband. It was also pathologising healthy mothers by keeping them in hospital for birth.

Antenatals were also where we co-planned a strategy for dealing with my terrible afterpains. It was not that my NHS midwives had been uncaring, but there was no time for anything outside core concerns – afterpains were not a core concern, so although they affected me enormously, they were never seriously discussed in terms of finding a solution. I just had to put up with it, and suffer it, in fact. With Michelle, we had a plan: there was homeopathy, there was acupuncture, there was shiatsu, there was bed rest.

There was, in a tactful and caring way, a discussion that can only happen between trusted people about not making things worse for oneself by worrying about it.

So we had a midwife who was truly professional and truly independent, who did her own research, who listened and had time for her clients, and who worked together with her clients for the best outcomes. She totally understood and worked within the paradigm of social care – the understanding that women's pregnant bodies don't come to clinic on their own, but are part of a woman with thoughts and feelings, who is part of a family and social network, all of which impact upon her, her choices, and her health and well-being.

The late great Mary Cronk, a well-respected independent midwife, left the NHS maintaining the NHS had changed and not her. She said:

"I worked in the NHS for thirty years, mostly in domiciliary practice – helping women have their babies at home in the way they wanted. I loved my job. I left in 1991 to start my own midwifery practice because it was becoming increasingly difficult to practice woman-centred midwifery within the NHS." [16]

The difference between an NHS midwife working for the hospital-based maternity services bound by their policies, and an independent professional working for me and my family, was massive. For a start, no consultant now had the right to tell a healthy woman that "only whales and dolphins have babies under water" and insist that his midwives ask me to leave the pool, just because he could.

Why did it take me so long to contact an IM since it was the maternity care that so suited my needs? During my fourth pregnancy at a meeting with the community midwifery manager (I can't remember why, maybe it was for the water birth 'talk'), I complained about the deterioration in the levels of midwifery care since my first birth. She told me that what I was wanting was a kind of care that they could no longer deliver and suggested that I contact the local independent midwives. We had so little money, I barely contemplated it. My husband was an archaeologist and archaeologists are poorly paid.

With baby no. 5, even with a discount, the cost of independent midwifery care was almost 20% of our then income and it took two years to pay off the debt! But it was so worth it. **So** worth it: to have someone who shared your values but had the expertise to deliver them, who gave you impartial information, had time to listen and discuss your concerns thoroughly, who knew so much because she researched so much, who had your back in a tight spot, and on the birth day would sit quietly in the room and not overtly intervene without necessity. I am convinced that Stan's birth (baby no. 4) would have gone differently with Michelle as my midwife.

We now have evidence via *The Lancet* papers[17] and the Cochrane Reviews[18] to show that continuity of midwifery carer throughout pregnancy, birth and beyond has a positive impact on mothers' and babies' experience of pregnancy, birth and the postnatal period. It is beneficial in reducing anxiety, worry and depression during the antenatal period. It reduces Caesarean sections, instrumental births and increases physiological birth. There is a lot of research around perception of pain, breastfeeding and postnatal depression being done and the picture is changing all the time as the research base develops. There is evidence around positive midwifery satisfaction and lower costs of maternity care.

If the maternity system implemented its own rhetoric of 'evidence-based medicine', then every woman in the country would have a midwife they knew and trusted. It does not, because the vested interests in the system do not gain in such an implementation, and those vested interests are powerholders. Community midwives and the women they care for are not powerholders in the system. I cannot emphasise enough that the lack of continuity of midwifery carer is **not** about money, it is about power. It is about the interests of those who hold the power and the purse strings. Midwife Professor Lesley Page CBE, along with others, has commented pointedly that if continuity of midwifery carer was a drug, everyone would have been prescribed it by now.[19]

Birthing Number 5 (Before the School Run!)

I was fed up. I was having strong contractions early each morning but they faded away by 7 am. It was Monday, five days after my 'due date'. I had decided to take up a suggestion from someone on my network, and wrote the question "What is stopping me going into labour?" on a piece of paper and put it under my pillow. I woke up the next morning with the blinding revelation that I was not going into labour… because of the school run! My husband worked away most weeks for 10 years, so I was conditioned to take the children to school, no matter what. Come 6.50 am and 2.50 pm, no matter how I was or what I was doing, I would be doing the school run.

My husband might be around in the week now but that conditioning was totally embodied, and my body was not going to birth a baby when the siblings needed to be taken to school. I therefore realised that this meant I would have to birth my baby either between 8.30 pm (when the children went to bed) and 6.50 am when I must rise to take them to school, or between 9.30 am and 2.50 pm (during the school day). The latter was too much pressure. I groaned: this meant a night birth.

Armed with this information, we planned my birth for the following day which was a Tuesday. The pool was filled, and I got in at around 8 pm; my husband joined me at 8.30 pm once the children were settled. We cuddled and canoodled to stimulate the oxytocin that would initiate the labour. Once those contractions were getting strong and regular, we rang Michelle, then I went into the kitchen to make myself a warm drink and slice of toast before we cracked on with the birth. Michelle had a very different view of a woman giving birth to her fifth child(!) and so she rushed over at once, arriving 20 minutes later.

We rang the film crew to let them know I was in labour. Oh, did I mention that my birth was being filmed for the *Desperate Midwives* documentary? But... they were having their Christmas party in Derby!

"I am so sorry! You should have told me! If I had known, I would have had the baby tomorrow night instead...!" I said.

Josh Whitehead, director and cameraman, had not come across women who called the shots on when she was having her baby. Anyway, he set off from Derby, and it would take him two hours to get to the house. Michelle, my husband and I had a council of war; we needed to halt the labour to give time for the crew to arrive. Oxytocin, the hormone of love, initiates and enables labour. Adrenalin, the hormone of stress, halts labour – it was the adrenalin that had been halting my labour every school morning. We needed to depress the oxytocin by raising adrenalin levels. So my husband was banished from the living room, we turned on all the living room lights and, bouncing on my birth ball for comfort, we engaged in loud and noisy conversation to engage the frontal cortex. Michelle knew how to press my buttons so she asked about the latest local maternity politics to raise my adrenalin levels! By the time Josh and his team arrived breathless at our door, cameras at the ready, my contractions had stopped.

"We thought you were going to have your baby!" he exclaimed.

"You did not want me to have the baby before you arrived," I responded calmly, "so we stopped the labour."

My husband and I scooted upstairs to our birth haven to resume the oxytocin stimulating cuddles, leaving Michelle to explain the mechanics of birth and how we manipulated them for their benefit. Within 45 minutes, the contractions were coming regularly and strong. Michelle crept in, followed by the cameraman and sound woman, careful to maintain that sense of darkness, quiet and privacy. Duke Ellington, Fats Waller and Doris Day were singing quietly in the background as I danced and moved through each contraction resting back into my husband's arms in between. Time went by: Jeanie arrived, and the children woke up and wandered in to find out what was happening.

"Do you want to watch *Bananas in Pyjamas*?" one of the adults asked.

Did they! At 4 am, this was a one-in-a-million chance! Jeanie took them downstairs and the strains of the video drifted up. Time went by and I was in transition: Did I want to be in the pool or did I not? Did I want to go to the toilet or did I want to birth a baby? Did I want to give up and go to sleep, or get the job done? And that music was annoying me!

In the end I gave birth standing in the pool, to Doris Day singing *Love Me or Leave Me*; apparently the team had it on repeat for 30 minutes because they observed it was the song this tired soul rallied for. I was deep in labour land, I had no idea! When my son birthed, he did so in one contraction, to everyone's surprise including mine (no crowning, head, then body stuff like normal). He was caught by several pairs of hands, and then was slowly, with much laughter, disentangled from the placenta cord – the cord was wrapped around his neck three times!

It was 6.40 am so there was plenty of time to get the children to school!

My final memory of the birth was bathed, snuggled in bed with baby in my arms, my husband asleep next to me, feeling like a million dollars, ringing any or everyone I could think of to share the good news.

Postnatal care started the same day. And it is only when you get proper postnatal care that you realise what an enormous difference it makes. I had daily visits for a week. And these were not 'check your vitals, check your stomach, then rush off to the next client, type visits, but drink a cuppa, talk through what happened, how you are now, how the family are, and so on.

By the end of the week, I was saying, "Please don't feel you have to come anymore. I have had more care in seven days than the previous three children put together! I don't need it like I did last time."

Most of my NHS community midwives apologised for the postnatal care; they knew it was not good enough at two or three often quite perfunctory visits in 10 days, then discharge. Thereafter, there were visits every other day or three times a week; postnatal care was for six weeks, not 10 days! But Michelle knew my/our history of postnatal depression and had determined it was not going to happen on her watch, so she did not discharge me for three months. She would ring me regularly – always on a day I was trying to do too much (yes, I am self-employed and yes, I started working as soon as I could feed and use a laptop at the same time!). In this way, she coaxed and coached me and our family out of danger; for that, I am ever grateful. Kindness as a profession – surely there is not a better one.

Sadly, such professionals are persecuted by NHS Trusts and the registration body (NMC) alike, so very few can now operate. Both mothers and midwives lose out. Michelle left independent midwifery to train midwives, and then left that to support women in other ways. Even from outside the NHS system, UK maternity is a brutal place to work in.

The Moral of This Tale – A Manifesto for Change:

In my life as in many others, continuity of midwifery carer from a midwife you know and trust made an enormous difference to the health and well-being of me (the mother) AND my family. This experience made me passionate and committed to ensuring every mother had continuity and personal care from a midwife within a small team – a passion and commitment that went even further than water birth because it was fundamental to the well-being of mothers and families.

Not every woman or birthing person needs the kind of care I needed. Different mothers have different social and emotional needs, BUT mothers and babies NEED the investment of one-to-one midwifery care in order to remain healthy, to care and guide them when they are not, and to help us 'pick up the pieces' and to carry on if it all goes horribly wrong.

Having real continuity of carer from a midwife I know and trust made me realise what a massive difference it makes to one's physical, mental and emotional health. It is a game-changer; it puts the odds in favour of making it through, even when things are bleak. I know that a midwife could not wave a magic wand and give us the money to fix the car and pay the bills, and they could not give my husband paternity leave or bring him home from working away.

But what they did was bridge the gaps of the understanding and skills I needed, gave us information, empowered us, gave us emotional and social support. Their support gave me the strength and confidence to carry on and not give up when the going got tough; they reminded me to give myself a break, take it easy.

They got me to a place where my social network could take over, and we two parents could stand on our own four feet.

If we invest in real continuity, real mother/midwife relationship care, if we take the needs of mothers seriously enough to ensure it happens, we will be investing in the health and well-being of not only mothers and babies, but also their families and their communities. It makes that much of a difference. I am testimony to that.

An Activist Born

This is my story; how I was 'woken up' to a failing inhumane system, how I learnt to survive it and navigate it to get the best care I could.

My story also demonstrates what good maternity care looks and feels like: it is personal, relationship-based, puts women and birthing people at its centre, not the system, and it is kind, always kind, and respectful. In this story, we have an ordinary mother without status or power (beyond her education and her colour) empowering herself within the system but also vulnerable to it. In liberation terms, this mother was 'conscientised' – that is, she became aware of the injustice and its systemic causes and was then motivated to change it: because I deserved the best midwifery care and so did my friends. And I believed I could make a difference by doing whatever I could do.

That is my story. You may have a similar story to tell. But now in Part 2, let us see what we as friends, siblings and allies can do about it; we can disrupt unhealthy patterns, challenge hurtful practices, and change attitudes and systems that harm mothers and midwives alike.

Part 2

~◦~

Being a Birth Activist

Chapter 5

～

Vision Into Action

SOME OF US BECOME activists to save our school, or sort out particular issues in our lives and situations, but then return to 'normal' life. Some of us make commitments to certain charities, community groups or political parties, and work through them. Others set boundaries on what we are prepared to do: collections at a supermarket or organise a fundraising event or editing the newsletter. I know women who, as a result of their experience and maybe some training, have gone on to ensure that their organisation has a breastfeeding policy or their clients get better breastfeeding information and support. All of these and other forms of activism are perfectly normal and acceptable and one is not better than the other: after all, we have different lives and choices.

For us to change the way the political wind is blowing, change needs to happen at many different levels and contexts in society. So you don't have to be an activist like me; you just have to be an activist like you. Ready to say that one thing that might help someone else, doing the one thing you can do. Everything that you do and say makes a difference. This book is about helping you to find your passion, and to give you some tools to make changes. Every change, big or small, is a change that makes the world better. The book is about giving you some ideas and showing what is possible; the rest is up to you!

Nonetheless, to understand the depth of my experience and expertise, it is important to know something of where it comes from and why. I did not set out to be a birth activist; I was already an activist and a social entrepreneur. I simply took this vocation and these skills into the birth arena. The work grew organically and exponentially over the years. I am still an activist but now I do it much more slowly!

I remember an ARM conference where the wonderful midwife Caroline Flint gave a keynote address telling the story of the beginning of the ARM. She talked about the first members taking a vow to talk every day to someone about midwifery and to someone about home birth.

She delighted the audience with stories of conversations at the supermarket checkout that began, "I need a lot of tea, you know. I am a midwife, you see, and we drink a lot of tea…"

I laughed, but thought: *I did not take a vow but I have been doing something similar for years.* At the school gates and toddler groups, I was talking about breastfeeding; at business meetings, I was eliciting (I don't know how!) the birth stories of everyone present, including all the men, and explaining what a good birth could be to anyone who would listen. I could be found lying down on countless carpets with the dog hairs to demonstrate how to breastfeed lying down. On one famous occasion, I was observed by our bookkeeper lying on the floor of our office talking through the breastfeeding technique with a woman – over the phone!

And the important thing to understand is that although it could be exhausting, I loved it; it was total fun! I don't think you can survive if you don't also find it fun: activism has to be energising for it to be sustainable. I also discovered I was an excellent grassroots strategist, a phenomenal networker and good at speaking out in public.

Supporting Breastfeeding

I not only ran a business but was also a lactivist – a term used for breastfeeding activists or sometimes just breastfeeding mums, in the days when mothers could be asked to leave a cafe or church, or moved from their seat whilst travelling for breastfeeding! I picked up the reins again with a son (child no. 5) at six weeks old in early 2005, interviewing for £60K funding for the nappy laundry service which launched in April the same year (which involved recruiting staff and so on). In 2005, I became one of the first breastfeeding peer supporters to be trained in Bradford and became an exponent (to any professional who would listen and anywhere I could write about it) of the strategic importance of embedding breastfeeding knowledge and skills in communities. Healthcare professionals (HCPs) are not and cannot be part of every community and be there whenever they are needed. Every street needs a person with knowledge and skill to whom people will turn. I saw breastfeeding peer support as a strategy to change baby feeding cultures: providing the information, support and nurturing to make that happen on the ground and in organisations and businesses everywhere in Bradford, in every language and accent. I was even one of the few laypeople who trained to become a breastfeeding peer support trainer and I helped set up two La Leche League mother-to-mother breastfeeding support groups – one of them in my home.

Later, via the MSLC, I occasionally attended the strategic breastfeeding group. Ideally, I wanted some of the local breastfeeding leaders to be part of the group rather than me. Firstly, I could not be everywhere at once and survive; secondly, for breastfeeding strategies in Bradford to work, they had to be collaborative – professionals cannot do it alone and neither can mums.

However (and I came up against this in so many of these strategic groups), we women/parents are usually the only unpaid person or persons there – the group is usually set up and structured by professionals at times and places convenient to them. For many breastfeeding mums like me, activism comes on top of a heavy workload of family commitments and day job. If, on top of the hours you spend on a support group, you must attend a strategic meeting that expects you to also find childcare and does not fit in with the school day, it fast slips down the priority list. Maybe the Zoom era should enable better participation of parents in strategic groups such as this.

> **Action Point: If you want to attend a change-making meeting, but cannot be there in person, ask to be able to attend via an online platform such as Zoom.**

And it's a shame, because I witnessed breastfeeding mothers being powerful and effective in strategic meetings when they were enabled to do so. As a peer supporter and then an active member of La Leche League, I went to a number of enrichment days (CPD, or training days with a better name!) and La Leche conferences. There was no arranged paid-for on-site childcare. I was told: "We just make sure there is a great sound system and plenty of space!" Mothers like me turned up to the conference with babes they were nursing plus older siblings, and they brought snacks and toys and set up shop over two or three seats perhaps. I had Tom at the breast, Stan or Tilly playing on the floor, and a notebook and pen on the chair next to me. These conferences attracted major speakers, and major pieces of medical research were presented. They were presented in a room full of mothers doing what they normally did – caring for their children whilst doing something else at the same time. And we did it!

It was so empowering to demonstrate to yourself and others you could do it all, to not feel you must apologise to anyone for your kids just being kids, and that you could absorb and participate in high-level discussion whilst caring for your children. I think the only reason mothers with children don't participate in strategic meetings is because the culture of maternity is all wrong. If we start with the mother and her children and structure from there, we would be able to participate strategically, no problem!

Action Point: Want to attend a meeting but need to bring your kids? Talk to the meeting organisers about a play area or space to have your children next to you at the meeting.

The breastfeeding peer support scheme was cut, of course, with the ending of Sure Start Children's Centres. It is part of the short-sighted attitude surrounding all maternity care that is more willing to invest large sums of money to deal with the health impacts of not breastfeeding/having a physiological birth, than invest the relatively small sums required for low tech information and support that preserves health and physiology. And because I can and always do(!), I have to add (as I always do) that not breastfeeding costs the NHS money. Not breastfeeding has been calculated as costing the NHS millions of pounds a year in treatment costs for diseases otherwise avoided from such as eczema and digestive problems, to diabetes, heart disease and breast cancer.[20] Notably, and to our shame, we have some of the lowest breastfeeding rates in Europe. The NHS maternity system in the UK is stupid!

The Choices Group (2002–2016)

The Choices group – set up about six months after the birth of baby no. 4 and which met in my home – was the foundation of my activism. After no. 5 was born, midwife Michelle insisted I had a break from hosting it for a few months. So began several years of nomadic life, sometimes meeting at my house, sometimes meeting in the homes of others – often women who had benefited from Choices themselves. When Michelle left, another independent midwife took over. Jo was such a different character but once in her stride, her humour and her down-to-earth attitude made her a star. Some couples came once or twice, some came right through pregnancy and beyond.

Here are a couple of examples of the difference these groups could make:

A woman came to the meeting for the first time. We started with introductions as usual: your name, where you might be in terms of pregnancy, what you want for your birth. When it came to her turn, she burst into tears. She had wanted a home birth for her first baby but it had all gone wrong, and that day she had been told she could not have a home birth this time either. And so it began, first with empowering information from Michelle, and second with an email to the consultant midwife explaining the situation and asking her to take the case on. When I sent an email like that, it was not the end of the matter; I would follow it up with the Trust and the woman to ensure an outcome that the woman was happy with, and everyone knew that. There were bumps in the road along the way for this particular mother, but one day I received a phone call from an ecstatic mum who had birthed her baby at home – she had done it! And she did it because we gave her information, and emotional and practical support, and we backed her up so she did not have to demand the care she wanted alone.

> **Reflection Point: As a birth advocate, the key is to support women to find their own power, or as much of it as they're ready to take on. Giving emotional support and information is the most**

empowering thing that we can do. However, doing the work for others can mean we inadvertently lead a woman down a path she does not want, but is not confident enough to say so. It is very important, therefore, to work *with* women rather than *for* women.

Another mum started coming when she was not pregnant and *after* her second baby was born. This was unusual but she was coming, she explained, as part of her PTSD therapy. She had been told her baby was too big and so had to be induced early. This resulted in a long and protracted labour ending in a C-Section. The baby born was not big at all. She was traumatised and angered by the experience. She had been lied to and she was angry at what had been stolen from her. She came every month to learn all she could. Often it would confirm to her how poor her previous care had been, and she understood what had not been done right. However, it also taught her the information she needed to make different choices, and the way to get them. She also knew we would back her up. In the end, she chose to freebirth (birth without a midwife present) because she felt she could not trust the maternity system to not do the same thing as last time and she could not afford an independent midwife. We supported her, not because we advised it, but because it was her right and her decision.

By the time this mum's fourth child came along (!), she was a stalwart of Choices and a valued host. The fantastic One to One Midwives team was in operation in Bradford at that time, headed up by a former independent midwife, and she was able to gain the mother's trust by providing the kind of care I received from my IM, Michelle. By her fifth child, she was a strong, knowledgeable and confident parent who could handle having the NHS midwifery team around. A listening ear, impartial evidence-based information, support and back up all the way – this is what we were able to offer through Choices.

> **Reflection Point: As advocates, people we support may choose options that we might not choose ourselves; supporting those choices is as important as supporting choices we may feel more comfortable with.**

As the years went on, there was an introduction into a network of birth workers, activists and midwives who turned to each other for support and mentoring.

The news of Choices spread and as more people benefited, other groups were set up in the region, some called Choices, some not. I collated them into my reminder email that now was a major newsletter. I no longer had the time to do it all and ended up paying for help. This is how a succession of talented women came into my office to research and write about birth – or turn what I was saying into copy.

Being a Social Entrepreneur

You have to understand that running our businesses and making them successful was part of my activism. I needed a living, and I needed a living that kept me independent of the system so I could not be sacked or put under financial or similar kinds of pressure. I needed a living because we had five children and they don't eat grass! This is an important point because some people employed in the public and voluntary sector do not always grasp this. Finally, one way to change the way the wind was blowing was to build a successful business providing maternity services women needed but were not currently provided – like birthing pools, cloth nappies... and baptisteries?

Aquabirths Birthing Pool Hire grew fast in those first couple of years; we went from 6 pools to 14 pools in 12 months. Meanwhile, our far-seeing business advisors pressed us to diversify to build the long-term stability of the business – and I hit upon a nappy laundry service like the one I had enjoyed when my first child was young. It was cloth nappies without any of the work. It was the convenience of disposable nappies without the carbon footprint and the waste going to landfill. It was to be a social enterprise and I obtained funding, business training and support. It was hard work though, to get the figures to stack up, the logistics sorted and apply for funding.

Then I became pregnant with Tom, my fifth baby. It was a business disaster! What I salvaged from it was the determination that I would use my pregnancy and birth in any way I could to promote water birth, good birth and cloth nappies, up to and including giving birth on TV – which is what I did. I interviewed for the funding for it when Tom was six weeks old in April 2005 and the Nappy Train was launched later the same year.

Nevertheless, whilst preoccupied with baby no. 5 and the start-up of the nappy laundry service, a new product and a new competitor came to market: offering cheap inflatable pools to buy. My pools were high-quality, hard-sided padded and insulated pools with robust quality equipment. A lot of my market saw it as a no-brainer: buying an inflatable that could be used for more than one birth. You could share it around, and it would double as a paddling pool for the kids, compared with a pool to be hired each time (however good the service), even if you never used it for birth. Inflatable pools also fit easily in the back of midwives' cars so are perfect for midwife supported home water births. The market profile had changed; I was focused elsewhere so there was nothing I could do about it, and we moved our business forward in other directions. From an activist rather than a business perspective, I might say the project had achieved its goal: I had provided birth pools for women in Yorkshire when there was no alternative. Now there was a cheap and affordable alternative, I could move on.

With cloth nappies, I moved from being the pool lady to the poo lady! What I discovered was that whilst women found it quite difficult to enter a conversation about home water births which combined two (healthy, evidenced) choices not supported by many local maternity services at the time, everyone was willing to talk about nappies! So many women approached me to talk about cloth nappies and then the conversation would move on to birth choices and breastfeeding. It was a gateway. Several customers came to see me about cloth nappies and were invited to Choices. Here they learnt about all the actual choices they had for birth, ended up hiring an independent midwife or doula, and having a home water birth in one of our pools using one of our little birth kits of complementary remedies and finished up attending a local breastfeeding support group or La Leche League and using cloth nappies or a nappy laundry service. However they entered the birth network, they benefited in terms of information, choice and support. Some went on to be doulas, breastfeeding supporters and counsellors, antenatal teachers, activists and so on, spreading the love, knowledge and empowerment, and doing far more than I ever could.

There were some in the public and voluntary sector who did not approve of these blurring of lines between the voluntary, public and private sectors; indeed, I personally had a hard time from some such people reducing me to tears. However, although I understand the fears expressed, my opinion is that in a healthy community ecology, these interrelationships occur naturally, and as long as they are not exploitative, are transparent, supportive and good. For me, personally, this was about information and choice – I would do almost anything to ensure women were able to make real effective choices – even setting up a business to provide it.

When the Nappy Train was running out of funding, I realised I needed to be strategically canny to ensure both the survival of the business and a continuing income for our family. So we did two things: set about building a sustainable future for the Nappy Train and then in tandem, looked for another sustainable income line for ourselves.

To build a sustainable future for the Nappy Train, we hosted a day conference inviting all of the region's nappy laundry services to discuss future sustainability and cooperation. At the end of the day of discussions, all but one laundry service decided to work together. The largest and oldest service delivered the service (collecting, washing and delivering the cloth nappies), and the rest of us would build the customer base and set up the first delivery. I worked like a Trojan to build our customer base and lobby our local authority, because we needed mass participation for long-term sustainability. We also needed support from the local authorities: we were delivering tons of reduction of landfill per baby and what we needed was a slice of the money saved to cover the set-up costs for each household. What killed us in the end was the cash flow – the set-up of new customers took money from the business and we did not have the resources to cover the cost until the babies made us money back. This was where we needed a public subsidy of £1-2K per customer to cover the initial outlay – but it was not forthcoming.

The death knell was an awful 2005 report that came out of the Environment Agency.[21] It was another travesty of evidence to the same degree as Bradford's water birth policy. Its conclusion was that there was no difference between using disposable and cloth nappies in terms of carbon footprint and that nappy laundries were worse for the environment.

You had to dig deep and read the appendices to learn, for instance, that this was based on households using old-fashioned terry nappies, that a third of users washed at 90 degrees – even nappy laundries did not do that! It was assumed that 10% of parents ironed their nappies too! There was also an assumption that nappies would not be used for a subsequent child.

For the uninitiated, we recommend washing at 40-60 degrees and line-drying. No ironing required! Our nappy laundries washed at 70 degrees for 10 minutes. Also, terry nappies are outdated – the world has moved on since my mother's time and there is a nappy style to suit every lifestyle! And finally, who throws away perfectly good nappies to spend another £200 on more for their next child!

Whatever its faults, the report ended any chance of getting public money to support cloth nappy use, let alone a nappy laundry. It was updated in 2008 and again in 2023[22], with much more realistic/accurate sets of assumptions. It is no surprise, therefore, that now cloth nappies are better for the environment than disposables! But too late for the nappy laundries...

When the end came, it was sudden. In a call from the guy running the logistics at 10 pm one night, we were told the business was closing then and there... Just to make it clear how social enterprises work, I should say we lost £12K of our own money, not to mention hundreds of hours of unpaid time, neither of which our family could afford. This was Monday 17th December 2007: the Nappy Train was three years old and so was my youngest son.

The Moral of This Tale:

Running a business or a social enterprise, or running an existing business in a particular way, is a form of activism. Like any form of activism, it has risks and costs, and you have to face the possibility of failure as well as success.

Baptistry UK

Meanwhile, we were looking to open another income stream for ourselves. As the competition from inflatables in an already competitive market made expansion of birth pool hire less feasible, we decided to go up a level and start selling birthing baths into NHS maternity units. We found an innovative bath manufacturer in Bradford and we were introduced to Mick, a master bath maker and designer who can make a beautiful bath from a sketch on the back of an envelope.

It took three years to break into the NHS market – the NHS is notoriously difficult to sell into. What finally helped us find our way in was the purchase of a competitor: we now had a history of selling birthing baths into the NHS! When we looked at the accounts of the business – and one has to pause to acknowledge how far we had come since we bought Aquabirths that we *actually* looked at accounts and did our due diligence! – it was clear that the most profitable part of their birth pool business was the baptistry hire!

For the uninitiated, the baptistries we are talking about here are not like the little stone fonts in Anglican churches, but large pools in which an entire adult is immersed as part of the ritual. Early in 2007, we bought the baptistry hire business, and also the installed permanent hospital birth pool business with the money that my Grandpa had left me, topped up by every penny of our savings. The rest went on the credit card.

Bearing in mind what was happening to the Nappy Train, you might imagine our situation. For about nine months, I gave up using cash machines to withdraw money because it seldom worked. If I had cash, I spent it on food and essentials; if I did not, we ate what was in the cupboard or in the freezer or did without. My husband was a financial whizz, robbing Peter to pay Paul, moving money around credit cards and bank accounts to ensure our mortgage and essential bills were paid, until the business began to turnover enough money to start paying ourselves something.

I wish to expunge from my memory the horror of that first Easter! In the following years, we streamlined and expanded the baptistries and kit we hired, worked on improving the logistics. We moved into sales of portable baptistries and equipment, and what took off was working with our bath manufacturer to build installed baptistries alongside our installed birth pools.

There were many challenges but the business grew, doubling in size every year for five years. The baptistry side of our business became two-thirds to three-quarters of our turnover, but significantly, my heart and soul was always with Aquabirths. But even that is not right: my heart and soul wanted women to have quality maternity care and real choices for birth (with or without water). The baptistry business and Aquabirths literally subsidised my obsession with ensuring quality maternity care and good birth for every woman.

Some Truths About Me and the Businesses

I was never profit orientated, although I could turn my mind to it when I needed. This meant, on the one hand, I had a vision and a goal that every unit and then every birthing room had a birth pool so ANY woman could have a water birth if she wanted one. It was a good business goal. However, on the other hand, I spent as much time as I possibly could on my passion to ensure every woman received quality maternity care and access and support for her birth choices. Remember, we had five children, we had three or more business lines, I was running the monthly Choices group and the growing network coming from it, I was hosting a monthly La Leche League in my home, I was Chair of the MSLC, and because I realised that national policy was affecting local decisions, I was networking nationally. From 2009, we also lived and worked in a dilapidated Victorian villa that needed doing up. Could I keep all those plates spinning?

Well, I did pretty well for several years. However, the business nearly went under at one point because I was too focused on my mission and did not keep a close enough eye on the balance sheet, which is crucial to managing an effective business.

The business was saved, thanks to an incredibly astute staff member, Heidi, who did some financial work and showed me the figures, helped us set up a recovery plan and then left because we could not afford her! This was July, and the recovery plan was that I had to sell five baptisteries per month for three months to ensure we could continue to trade. I turned my phenomenal energy to saving the business and sold three baptisteries in a week and then hit the three-month target in a month. However, I had learnt my lesson: my passion for good birth should not absorb my attention so much that I lost sight of practical living. I had to reduce the hours I spent on the MSLC and other unpaid work.

There were consequences. For instance, I could no longer attend the Maternity Services Management meeting on a Monday morning (ffs!!!) which was basically the MSLC without the invitation to lay people. I was the only service user representative invited but Monday was the busiest day for the business: I could not go. This meant I missed input into important discussions, missed out on information sharing and so on. I tried to find a way for someone else to attend on my behalf but it was 'not possible'. In turn, this had major consequences when difficulties arose later on.

The MSLC (2007–2013)

The Maternity Services Liaison Committee (MSLC) was then called the MVP (Maternity Voices Partnership), now called the MNVP (Maternity and Neonatal Voices Partnership).

This story began after I had asked my first question at the Trust's AGM. I had been regularly writing with my concerns about maternity care to the CEO of Bradford Trust: he had given me his card at the AGM where I asked my first question, suggesting that I contacted him rather than the press. A new Head of Midwifery had been appointed, Julie Walker. She was one of the team of community midwives who had supported me after my first birth. She had told this weepy mother that I was doing okay, that I was a caring mother even if I did not feel like one (I did not understand then how trauma works so you don't feel anything), that mums often felt this way, but she could see the baby was healthy and looked after, and so on. I will never forget her kind and encouraging words.

A few days after she was in post, one of the first things she did was call me and invite me in for a chat. I had not been invited to any chat or consultation since my complaint! I cannot remember the conversation except that it was positive and that we agreed to work together.

I was then invited along to a meeting at a community centre to discuss the revival of the MSLC, a then statutory meeting that included all the stakeholders in maternity care and usually chaired by a layperson.

I came home from that meeting and said to my husband, "This is it! I know I have far too much on my plate but this is the most important and significant thing I could be involved in. I will do whatever it takes and clear the diary if necessary."

The thing was, Choices empowered women and we changed the system a little as we supported women to make their choices and the maternity system accommodated them, if grudgingly sometimes. But here was an opportunity to make changes at a strategic level so women did not have to fight any more for things like a home birth, for a water birth, to decline some medical advice, to receive good continuity of midwifery carer, and so on.

When, after a few months we needed a new chairperson, there was that usual pause, no one else stepping forward. I said I would do it. Julie had laughed a few months earlier when I commented in a meeting that the best way to stop me being a troublemaker was to give me a job – and now I had a job.

At the final MSLC meeting I chaired, Julie told us the very beginning of this tale: When she was appointed as Head of Midwifery, she was called to a meeting with the CEO of the Trust (the one I had been writing to and asking questions of at AGMs!). He gave her my card and said "Deal with THAT woman!" And she did. She gave me a job to keep me out of trouble…!

The MSLC and the Bradford Birth Centre

The Birthplace Cohort Study[23] surveyed nearly 65,000 births in low-risk women across the UK in all settings. What it found was that birth was safe for women and babies WHEREVER the birth takes place. However, the chances of having a physiological birth was 87.9% at home, 83.3% in a free-standing birth centre, 76% in a hospital birth centre, and only 57.6% in a hospital delivery suite or obstetric unit.

Similarly, C-section rates in the healthy low-risk group were almost four times higher for women giving birth in an obstetric unit. Bradford had nearly 6,000 births at this time with the vast majority being born in the delivery suite. If you did not want this hospital birth, the only option was a home birth, not everyone's cup of tea. Women on the Calderdale side of Bradford were popping across the border to birth in their birth centres, so much so that there was apparently a row over who should be paying. Bradford needed a birth centre.

The birth centre was not my brainchild but, in partnership with the senior midwifery team, it was certainly our shared goal. There was much mutual support and consultation, and not solely about the colour of the walls (frequently the only thing women are consulted on!). The lead appointed for making it happen was Deborah Hughes, a redoubtable and solid midwife leader. She was a former independent midwife and a community midwifery team leader who pioneered supported home water births and physiological birth at home after previous C-section (called VBAC conventionally). She had researched and written about why birth centres frequently failed[24]. She was recruited to ensure it did not happen to this one.

What worked so well was the dance that gave space for different stakeholders to do what they did best. The senior midwives were negotiating budgets and policies and we left them to it, but they came to the MSLC to ask us what we thought about this policy or that issue. If they were having difficulty getting something through, they shared this with us and asked for ideas, comments and opinions – drawing on that wider pool of information and knowledge, sometimes called 'the hive mind'.

We also gave them leverage to go back and say, "Women won't accept that". Where we, or indeed I, came into my own is when those negotiations stalled, or there was that great big silence when it was time for the Trust to commission and pay. I was able to write one of 'my letters' copied to all and sundry to provide that kick up the backside some institutions need to do the right thing – it was the same CEO so he knew my handwriting!

Alternatively, I might ask questions at a public conference or the AGM such as, "What is happening with the birth centre? Can you confirm it is going ahead as planned?"

I was told afterwards that these salvos across the bows of Trust pushed them back to honouring their commitment or returning to the table to take things forward.

In all, it took four years to get the birth centre off the ground, in which there were two budget cuts and a number of wobbly moments. But we managed it! We had three pools installed, the unit was a separate midwifery-led space with separate staff managed separately from the labour ward, and we had a separate entrance to the birth centre so women coming to the birth centre did not have to go via the Obstetric Unit. We had low lighting installed, gentle colours and non-institutional soft furnishings. We achieved a system where low-risk women would be offered the birth centre as a default – that is, if they did not express a preference for a place of birth, this was where they came. Incredibly, about one-third of babies born in the hospital were born in the birth centre in the months following its opening.

The Moral of This Tale:

- We pulled off this project because, as an MSLC, we pulled together as a team, across ideological and professional boundaries, working to each other's strengths and roles. Sometimes we were opponents, but on this issue, we were a team.

- If you don't stay 'on top' of an NHS Trust, they will try to slide out of investment in low-tech maternity care, even if it delivers great outcomes and is what women and midwives want.

- Often, simply asking a question in a public (or private) setting is enough to push a project forward. It also stops them from saying, "No one is asking for it"!

- 'Salvos across the bows' can help organisations honour their own aims and commitments too.

The MSLC and One to One Midwifery in Yorkshire (2011–13)

This next section was very difficult to write.

As Chair of the MSLC, I sometimes brought in speakers to widen horizons, give us new ideas, some blue-sky thinking and consider different ways of doing things. After my experience of continuity of carer throughout the maternal pathway with a midwife I knew and trusted, I was keen to see this being delivered to every woman in the district, most especially to those who needed it most. The unborn babies of the poorest women in Bradford were, according to the Born in Bradford research[25], significantly more likely to die than the babies of the wealthiest women in Bradford District. Overwhelmingly, deaths were concentrated in the South Asian community. Even today, infant mortality is way above the national average and concentrated in the South Asian population[26]. These were outcomes that, according to the evidence, could be improved with continuity of carer.

I invited various people who could give a window on how such care might be delivered, and how it was being delivered in other areas: people who could share experience and data on how continuity of midwifery could work. When I invited speakers, I would often introduce them into wider community networks, because the issues we were trying to solve were not going to be solved by the NHS alone. People and organisations in the community needed to understand both the problem and the potential for change – and in turn, they might be able to help. Indeed, the large infrastructure organisations in Bradford have, in subsequent years, intervened to provide the kind of maternity care their populations need. From the networks I was building nationally, I knew policies and guidance were coming down the line that could/would make this happen, and I wanted Bradford to be ahead of the curve.

To cut a very long story short, One to One Midwives – a private, midwife-owned, midwifery company offering continuity of carer services wholly funded by the NHS (like a GP practice) – decided to start operating in Bradford and West Yorkshire without the express invitation of the commissioners – mainly on the back of policies and guidance which enabled the funding for it. The commissioners and other stakeholders ignored my letters asking for meetings and discussions on continuity of midwifery carer for many months. With the emerging evidence about how continuity reduced rates of miscarriage, premature birth and stillbirth, it seemed a no-brainer for our communities where infant mortality was so high. But the system and many powerful people in it did not care enough, did not want the status quo challenged, and were going to hold off any change for as long as they possibly could. After I had some private conversations with senior managers in Bradford Maternity, I understood the challenges to implementation far better and had sympathy for their predicament.

However, these challenges were not insuperable: the same planning, determination, negotiation and perseverance that got us our birth centre could get us continuity of carer.

Action Point: Keep talking to those in power and understand their perspectives. Knowing the barriers they face helps you to work with them to find ways to overcome them.

Due to new government policies at the time, the commissioning organisations for healthcare were in transition, so there was a lack of communication and leadership, and warnings were missed. The commissioners (the organisation which holds and distributes NHS money locally) and some hospital managers said they were taken totally by surprise. They were shocked and angry that a midwifery practice wholly funded by the NHS in the same way as GP practices should come into their area with pregnant women and people self-referring into it, and midwives applying to work for it. One to One Midwives delivered the kind of midwifery midwives wanted to do and the kind of care women wanted to have – but how dare they! There were rows, and more rows.

Casting about for someone to blame, I was singled out: play the person, not the ball. Having refused to meet me to discuss continuity of carer as a vehicle for improving outcomes for the poorest women in Bradford, they suddenly wanted to meet me to discuss how I was acting outside my role, inviting One to One Midwives to speak at the MSLC on one occasion. I was accused of being paid by this private company to promote it!

I was then, and continue to be, totally nonplussed. I thought that, like me, surely everyone wanted to reduce infant mortality, improve outcomes for mothers and babies, especially the poorest, and deliver excellent evidence-based care within budget. So why was there so much opposition to a solution handed on a plate that cost them no more money? I have never understood.

Ten years on, having promised it could deliver this care without One to One Midwives, Bradford have still failed to do so, except for a small number of women. The best work has been achieved by one of the infrastructure organisations I talked with all those years ago. I am not singling out Bradford as one bad example because this was happening all over the country, demonstrating the systemic rather than personal nature of the issue: the maternity system is more interested in supporting itself than it is in delivering the care women need. The suffering that I had set out to prevent happening to anyone else is now a choice, not an inevitability.

This means, therefore, that the choice has been made that the suffering of mothers is **less important** than the maintenance of existing powers and interests. Pregnant and birthing people continue to be bolt-on extras to the main event.

The Moral of This Tale:

- This story demonstrates the lesson that when we stop working together, listening to and respecting one another, things fall apart, and mothers and families suffer poorer care.

- Here are the consequences of women and pregnant people not being at the centre of care: choices are not made for their benefit, but for the benefit of power holders within the maternity/ NHS system. This has happened time and again. This is just one representative example.

- We see that losing the strong voice of informed and empowered service users at the table where strategic decisions are made, negatively impacts maternity care. You cannot pay an MSLC Chair for four hours a week and expect her to be at every strategic meeting. Such paltry money, such paltry hours, shows a fundamental lack of recognition that the participation of informed and empowered service users and their representatives is fundamental to the delivery of the excellent care that mothers want and need. It also demonstrates a lack of respect.

- **When an institution feels under threat, it will find a scapegoat – preferably, but not necessarily, outside its ranks.**

The End of an Activist (Maybe?)

During this period, my health began to deteriorate. At the time, I was too busy to be aware. It was a case of feeling extremely tired; the high jinks and challenges were not fun anymore. I was losing heart and vision. I was breathless walking up mild inclines. I began to think of succession. I put in structures and sought out people so that I could slowly withdraw. I began to dream of living in a place where every encounter was not a conversation about birth. It was a long, slow process, perhaps taking about four years.

It was only when I was so ill that I could barely walk that I visited a doctor and discovered my iron level was half what it should be. Perimenopause had slipped in the back door, but I was too busy to notice what she was up to; I had just carried on dealing with the heavier periods and carrying on regardless.

My iron level returned to normal but my energy levels did not, and every time I picked up my pace of work, my iron levels dropped again. In the end, to recover and retain my health, I had to give up everything: working on the business, working on my passion for women to birth, activism of every kind.

Chapter 6

~

Holding to Account

THIS BOOK IS NOT A HANDBOOK to tell you how to make change happen, disrupt and protest. I want it to be a story that inspires and guides, with ideas, useful tips and tactics which you can adapt and use for your own situations. It is a 'passing on' of learning, experience and skills, as it was passed down to me by the activists I learnt from. What I hope you will see underlying these stories are strategies for holding organisations responsible for maternity care to account. We are not asking them to do anything they were not already signed up to – we are simply asking organisations to live up to their own standards and ethos.

All the stories that follow are inevitably cameos, and despite my efforts to paint some of the context, the complexities of the situations have to be omitted. So, use the stories as ideas and inspiration rather than a manual of what to do in every given situation. I am offering advice and pointers but your situation and position will be different; realise that for yourself, you will have to do it your own way.

As a budding social entrepreneur, I was taught that you can do all the research and all the planning you want, but in the end, it comes down to JFDI (JUST F****** Do It!). Ultimately as an activist, it is JFDI: you do your research, you do your planning, but in the end, you must simply jump in, do your best, and not worry that it might all go wrong (or do, but do it anyway!). Then work out what happens next, when what happens next has happened!

Researching a talk some years ago, I discovered a lovely story of a couple who had a disastrous start to their business. When asked by the interviewer if they had done ANY business planning, they answered "Yes. And it had three points: Have a go. See how it goes. Take it from there!" I would do some planning and research first, but in the end, that really is all you can do.

It Is Not the Answer, It Is Asking the Question That Matters

The first time I asked a question at an NHS Trust's AGM, I was shaking like a leaf, even though my independent midwife was sitting beside me to give me support. There were a hundred or so people in the room when the new Chief Executive asked for questions. I nearly missed my chance but my question was taken. I read out my question, carefully prepared beforehand, ensuring that the wording contained the medical evidence on which it was based.

It went something like: "According to medical evidence, women are half as likely to have a C-section if they book a home birth, even if they later transfer into hospital. In the light of this evidence, why is it so difficult for women in Bradford to book a home birth? Why is the home birth rate so low?"

I did not expect a coherent answer from the CEO since he had had no notice of the question and it was clear from the answer he knew little, if anything, about maternity. My strategy was to get the issue on the agenda. There were over 100 people, mainly women, listening to my question. The local media was present, and, of course, it would be in the minutes of the AGM. There was a buzz from my question – I had hit the spot!

As soon as the meeting finished, I saw the local newspaper reporter heading towards me. But – and all these years later, I still find this most amusing – the very sharp CEO had also spotted the reporter and came right across the room to intercept our meeting, introducing himself and commenting on the interesting question I raised.

We conversed for half an hour, during which I pressed my case using my experience and that of others at the Choices group I ran, and pointing to the principle of evidence-based practice in maternity care.

He closed the conversation by giving me his card and saying, "Contact me directly rather than going elsewhere if you have an issue."

Which, of course, I did. About every eight weeks...

The end of this story we now know: a few months later, the new Head of Midwifery was given my card by the CEO of the Trust and told her to "Deal with THAT woman!" And so she did, by asking me to be part of setting up the new MSLC.

The Moral of This Tale:

- **It is always worth asking a question at large formal meetings such as a Trust's AGM, Council Scrutiny committees, Consultation events, etc.**

- **The important thing to understand is that it is not the answer to your question that is crucial most of the time; it is the fact that you have asked it and raised the issue. You are putting it on the agenda.**

- **Always prepare the question beforehand. Even if it occurs to you during the presentation, jot it down if you can and get the wording right. I remember at a parliamentary committee saying I had prepared a question, and the Chair, Baroness Cumberlege commented, "Of course you have!" before asking me to proceed!**

- **Think about the point you want to make, the issues you want to raise and the best way to raise it in the question. Emotion can be powerful on occasion, but needs to be handled carefully. It is more important that the question is heard by your listeners than you to express your feelings.**

- Do not assume that the person answering, nor indeed the whole audience, knows what you are talking about. So, if possible, like me, fold a statement of evidence or fact into the question, or a short explanation from which the question is asked.

- You never know where a question might lead: a conversation with the CEO, an article in the local media, a place on a consultation. Asking a question often resulted in an interesting dialogue with someone useful or helpful.

- A supporter beside you can really help your courage levels. My independent midwife, being the fabulous midwife she is, seeing that I had succeeded in our strategy, melted into the crowd and disappeared.

Busting the Stone Wall

Sometimes you don't get an answer to your question, no matter how often you ask or how many different ways you try to raise the issue. This was the case during a large structural reorganisation of commissioning of healthcare taking place whilst I was chairing the MSLC. At each meeting, we would try and get some information: we would ask the maternity commissioner for updates, information or reassurances – different things at different meetings. She simply repeated what was clearly the line she was told to give.

We were being stonewalled. No one from the old or the new organisation would come to the meeting and tell us what was going on. When we requested contact with a decision-maker, we were given no name, and no one in either organisation would answer if I contacted them. We did not even know if there would be an MSLC in the new world being planned behind closed doors.

After several months of this, I came up with the following strategy: I used my extensive Bradford network to trawl for any information whatsoever, even rumour and gossip. I went to a Council for Voluntary Services Information Day for community groups on the transition from PCT to CCG (acronyms for organisations you no longer need to worry about!) where I discovered that the whole sector had received a similar line to us, but some people had succeeded in getting a little more detail than others. I collated everything I had from well-sourced information to frankly rumour and gossip into a formal briefing paper for the next MSLC meeting. It deliberately went out in the meeting papers in advance of the meeting. I presented it as the best knowledge the city of Bradford could offer in answer to the questions we had been asking each meeting.

I would have liked to have been a fly on the wall when that paper landed in the commissioner's office because at the meeting, the commissioner told us that the briefing was all inaccuracy and supposition – which, of course, it was! I was told that it should not have been shared with the MSLC without checking with the organisations first (but that was the whole point of the exercise!). She then went on to say that both the current and future commissioning organisations now recognised that there was an information gap being filled with rumour and misinformation (which was absolutely true!) and to counter that ... she proceeded to provide the basic information we had been asking for all along. It was all done with a certain amount of humour and twinkling of eyes because, of course, everyone knew what I had done, and also knew why.

The Moral of This Tale:

- **If you are being stonewalled and perfectly reasonable questions are going unanswered and emails and phone calls ignored, find a strategy to highlight this with lightness and humour.**

- **Sometimes, calling an organisation's bluff by presenting their own lack of information back to them in a very public way, can just do the trick.**

- **Even if you don't get the information you want, they are forced to justify their response in the public domain rather than the private, promoting transparency and accountability.**

This is holding to account, because public bodies are accountable.

Writing *the* Letter

Even today, letters are a fabulous tactic of campaign and change with a proven track record. Here are a few tips to make that letter work hard for you – because an effective letter will take a long time to draft, write and send, so it needs to be worth the effort.

- Address the letter to the highest authority possible in the organisation. Don't write to the Head of Midwifery (HOM), but write to the CEO of the Trust and copy it to the HOM. Don't write to the manager of an organisation, write to the CEO/owner and copy in the manager, and so on. As my husband puts it picturesquely, "Shit is rarely shovelled upwards: those at the top will ensure the shit always falls on those beneath."

- Even when expressing anger and a full helping of indignation, the letter should always be faultlessly courteous. You need people to take in what you are telling them, and they are less likely to do so if it is too angry and personal. In addition, it is often the case that the person you are writing to or even whom you are writing about, is not actually directly responsible for the complaint, even if they are the ones ultimately responsible for sorting it out.

- If we want kindness in our world, we need to emulate it in our letters, in our questions, in our meetings. Be forceful, but also be kind.

- Clearly and carefully set out the issue, problem or complaint, using examples, evidence and references as necessary. Bullet points can be your friend, especially with a long chronology, so that an uninformed reader can follow the steps of the problem and doesn't get lost in a long and difficult story.

- State clearly what you want the person to do. Make sure the key actions are within their authority (which is why it is worth starting from the top) and possible to accomplish in a reasonable amount of time. For example:

"We want the policy to be changed to allow partners to accompany women and pregnant people into every scan, or have the alternative of connecting with their partner via video call: a woman should not have to attend a sonography appointment alone where bad news may be learnt." This is clear, concise and doable. If a change of culture is required, then this can be stated, but stepping stones for progress need to be given. I may want the induction rate to drop significantly, but stepping stones along the way could be the publication of the audit on induction at the unit, appointing a manager to be responsible for reporting to the forum every month, investigating reports of coercion, the publication of a strategy with regular updates to ensure progress, and so on.

- A good letter takes a lot of time. My letters generally take four to seven days to write from start to finish. Research of evidence, collation of previous correspondence, checking timelines and so on, takes time and needs to be right. Draft, redraft and then sleep on it. Both wording and tone are important.

- Have another pair of eyes and a strategic head to read your letter if you can – someone who can soften a sharp phrase and sharpen a phrase that is too soft. In my case, a proofreader is also essential!

- Writing the letter is time-consuming and hard work, so don't undertake this kind of letter lightly or when you are pushed for time. Make the letter work for you by copying in everyone who is remotely relevant, but especially the key people in the sector, so not only can the CEO see who you have copied the letter to, but the other key players you have copied in will see who the CEO is. We want to ensure reputations are at stake.

- As Chair of the MSLC, I copied my letters to everyone on the MSLC mailing list, plus all the local MPs on my patch. If relevant, I would also copy to the CEOs of national organisations such as NCT, AIMS, ARM, RCM, and so on, *and* to the Chair of the Parliamentary Health or Maternity Select Committees etc. Spread the shit liberally and widely.

- Most important is copying in your MP. Have your MP (of whatever political colour) on side if you possibly can; brief them and cosset them because they will protect you from some of the personal stuff that could be thrown at you when organisations feel threatened.

- Also, if confidentiality is not an issue, copy it to your best media contacts. It can take a bit of work to collate all the contacts but, boy, is it both scary and fun to hit that send button!!

- And another thing. When you get the reply, or replies, whatever they are like, don't read them when you are tired and low. And whatever you do,

don't answer them right away. Let the words sink in because most official letters are written in code, and you need to work out what they are actually saying or offering, or sometimes what they are **NOT** saying underneath the organisation-speak. Seek out people who may help you decipher the code.

The Length of the Letter

The general rule of thumb is to keep your letter on one page, like a press release. Remember the principle of conciseness, ensuring that a reader does not have to turn the page to find out what the complaint is about. However, if the letter concerns complex issues and comes at the end of a protracted process to raise or resolve the matter, then it is unlikely the letter will be one page. As you see in the following example, my letter was in response to the Trust's 'final statement' on a controversial issue which I sought to demolish, so it was not going to be short! Nevertheless, ensure that if only the start and end of the letter are read (which maybe the case for those you copy in), the message is heard loud and clear. And try to ensure within the limitations of the letter form that the letter is a page-turner, with no waffle! Keep it moving!

The following letter is an example. The context is the beginning of the Covid-19 pandemic. It came to my notice through posts of fellow activists that pregnant women and people at Leeds NHS Teaching Trust were not allowed to have ANY support from their partner or supporter at their antenatal scan; not only were they not allowed to attend in person, but they were not allowed to connect via video link either! Up to 20% of women have bad news from a scan – including the death of their baby. There is a massive lack of compassion in preventing both parents or partners to be present at such news; there is even a legal argument that it is deprivation of the right to family life. On the then MVP's (now called MNVP) Facebook Forum, we asked the Trust for their reasons, then we challenged their reasons which were often superficial and did not make sense when scrutinised. We tried to negotiate wiggle room for women. We highlighted that mothers with disabilities, such as being deaf and blind, were being denied appropriate support, and so on. After several weeks of toing and froing, I had enough and decided to write one of my letters.

The Letter

Dear Julian,

I am writing to complain about the Trust's continuing policy towards the attendance of partners at maternity scans and video-calling at them. I also wish to complain about the statements put out by the Trust on the topic, which are frankly insulting to the many women who have read them. I will go through last week's statement in detail below.

Her story:

However, first, for you to understand the gravity of the situation, I wish to share a post by a mother about her scan:

Today I went in for my 10-week scan, alone. Due to COVID, spouses aren't allowed at your appointment which meant when the tech said, "I'm sorry, there is no heartbeat," I had to process that information, alone.

I had to get off the chair and collect my things in tears while nurses asked me questions I couldn't even comprehend.

I had to hold my composure and walk to another room alone to wait for the doctor to tell me what I already knew.

I had to sit alone in a room until they finally allowed my significant other to come inside.

How are we allowed to go shopping, drink at bars, and eat at restaurants, but I can't have support with me when someone tells me my baby is dead? That moment was absolutely soul-shattering and I had to do it alone, with no one to turn to because the clinic says, "Spouses cannot attend ultrasounds."

Today is a terrible day and it's one I'll never forget. Sadly, my significant other wasn't there to experience it so he will never fully understand what it felt like to look at our baby in real-time and see no heartbeat. I saw it, alone, and it was heartbreaking.

If I can shop, dine and drink, my significant other should be able to attend the appointment to see his child.

Rest in peace, little one.

This is not a game. This is not about beating those 'stroppy mums' who keep moaning and complaining; this is about the hearts and lives of mothers, fathers and their children. It is for this reason that I am particularly incensed by the latest statement which I quote in its entirety below, in case you have not read it. My complaint is detailed point by point below. Because of the seriousness of the situation, and the persistently poor and evasive responses from the Trust, I am copying this letter to key people across the maternity sector, to local MPs and national politicians with a remit for the sector. This matter needs to be resolved, but not in the manner the Trust is attempting at present. For a start, respect is required.

Trust statement:

"Following further discussions with LTHT and the Radiology department, we have been able to establish that there is legislation in place that allows patients to record consultations with their doctors. However, an ultrasound scan is considered a diagnostic test, not a consultation, and therefore considered differently. In line with guidance from The Royal College of Radiologists and other national professional societies, the Radiology department have advised that video recording of these appointments cannot be permitted. Reasons given for this decision relate to levels of distractions created by video-calling or recording and staff safety.

"Discussions have been had with other trusts across the country and the decisions within LTHT are in line with those at other trusts. Unlike many other trusts, LTHT have been able to ease restrictions on the attendance of partners at most scan appointments. As women now have the support of their partner, this should reduce any need to film the scan. Video capture/footage can be purchased through private scan providers, Radiology would not endorse or recommend any one specific provider.

"Unfortunately, having been able to clarify this point, the MVP have been advised that this is the final position of the Radiology department at this time. The MVP will continue to share comments in relation to this, however, have been made aware that this decision is unlikely to change in the near future.

"We sincerely apologise for this outcome, and can only advise those that are affected by this to make a formal complaint if they feel that their care has been affected by this decision. The MVP are able to support those who choose to do this."

Point-by-Point Complaint

1. Medico-legal reasons. We have still not been given medico-legal reasons strong enough to deny women their right to have support and to video call any consultation. Your statements so far do not bear scrutiny.

2. Diagnostic test. It is an interesting argument to say that the scan is a diagnostic test and therefore is exempt from the right to record or video call. Interestingly there are no definitions given but by my definition this would mean, therefore, that the woman is given NO information during the scan itself and the sonographer could answer no questions as to what is observed or measured. If they were to do so, the test immediately becomes a consultation. This means that at a placental placement scan, if the sonographer shows the woman where the placenta is, or at a growth scan if the sonographer communicates any measurements or concern, then the diagnostic test becomes a consultation and under the rules as stated above can be recorded.

3. Legal advice. In no legal advice we have read so far in the interests of patients has there been this discrimination between diagnostic and non-diagnostic consultations. The advice is to record all consultations overtly or covertly as necessary because both are admissible in court. There is NO legislation in place to deny women the right to record any consultation, diagnostic or not. Either the Trust needs to publish your lawyer's advice for all to see and scrutinise, or this should be rescinded.

4. Distraction. I think it is just that – a distraction. We have repeatedly asked precisely what is the difference between the distraction of a partner in the room which is acceptable, and a partner present via video link which is not. Due to this being about Covid-19 restrictions to prevent infection, we cannot understand why the Radiology department thinks it is safer to have a partner in the room than to have the partner attending via video link. None of the superficial reasons given early on (in June/July) stood up to any scrutiny – is this why we have no answer? This statement does not answer the question but repeats the word distraction without defining it. This is not good enough. And demonstrates the ongoing disrespect for our intelligence and the reasonable request of an honest answer to a straight question.

5. That the problem has gone away because partners are allowed to attend scans. The problem has not gone away because not all scans are accessible to partners and this has been raised and clarified on a number of occasions on both the MVP forum and on the E-Midwife group. It is in these scans that video recording is an essential tool to enable partners to fulfil their role as a parent and for women to receive the support they wish to have. If the restrictions tighten once more, then video calling is an essential fall-back position for women and, therefore, it is not acceptable to say the problem has gone away.

6. Paying for scans. To say in a forum concerning NHS care that women can purchase footage or scans as an alternative to being present at the scan consultation in reality or virtually, beggars belief in a Covid-19 pandemic where hundreds of families have lost their jobs and incomes. The Born in Bradford survey states that 1 in 10 of the parents said their food did not last and that they could not afford more (BBC News website).

7. Consultation with the Royal College of Radiology. In essence, this means the Trust has consulted with the Sonographers Union, a body set up primarily to promote the interests of sonography and its members. It is not primarily set up to represent the interests or needs of women and their families. For the Trust to state openly that it has consulted with the professional associations of sonographers, but not to have consulted with similar institutions representing women's interests such as Birthrights, the NCT, AIMS or even the National Maternity Transformation Programme Board, is astonishing. It clearly demonstrates a Trust that puts the needs of women and families in its care a poor second to the interests and idiosyncrasies of staff unions. It is at this point that I feel that I must live in a parallel universe where the NHS was set up to care for the health of the people in its care and is paid for, and accountable to the public – not to unions or professional associations, however august their names.

8. We are in line with other Trusts we have talked to. This looks very much like an organisation trying to justify itself by saying it is no worse than its friends. I am not sure I want to dignify this point with a response. Good practice and morality have never been based on what other people do, but on what is right, proper and appropriate. And indeed in a court of law, Leeds Trust would be answering for its own actions and not that of others.

9. Closing down the debate. I am concerned at the precedent this latest statement sets in terms of the Trust's relationship with the MVP. As I understand it, the MVP is a forum where the stakeholders in maternity care meet to discuss issues of interest to us all. The MVP is not the messenger for the Trust when it wants to close down an ongoing debate. I am disappointed that the Trust did not see fit to write its own statement to service users and the public, but asked the MVP to pass on the message. Presumably so that the MVP could take the flak and not the Trust because the Trust does not want to hear any more about the subject. This is not how democracy and accountability work. And I am disappointed that you put the MVP in such a position. Until a solution agreeable to all sides is found, then it is the duty of the Trust to continue to listen to the concerns of public and service users. You cannot unilaterally close down the discussion. I think an apology is in order here to the MVP for using them in this way and to those stakeholders who this statement has tried to exclude.

10. Making a formal complaint. This letter is in part a response to the invitation to make a formal complaint. However, I must inform you that another woman has made a complaint via PALS and the first response was to ask for her full name, her date of birth and her NHS number. She was incensed by this intimidatory behaviour and refused to provide the information and the request was withdrawn and an apology made. However, if this is the treatment women receive when invited to make a complaint on this matter to the Trust, I am appalled and I hope that you are too. Many women are already afraid that any complaint they make about their care may affect the future care they receive – this confirms that fear. As an addition to the Trust's responses so far, this demonstrates again a wholly unacceptable attitude to the women and families in your care, particularly anyone who expresses disagreement with policy. What I require is a formal apology to the woman concerned by the Trust, an enquiry into the handling of complaints by PALS, and the Radiology department to ensure this NEVER happens to anyone else. And I would like a statement on the MVP and E-Midwife Forums explaining clearly the complaints process and rights women and their families have within that. Finally, the statement should reassure women that they will be treated with respect and confidentiality throughout the process and beyond, with no repercussions for future care.

Conclusion:

I think the saddest part of this affair is the lack of compassion for women and their partners, and the unwillingness to work in partnership with us to find an acceptable solution in this time of crisis and restriction. The statement indicates a 'them and us' perception that sees those of us who criticise as 'them', and as a problem, rather than part of a team working together for the benefit of women and their families. This attitude must cease at all levels, especially in the sonography department if this issue is to be resolved without more upset.

Actions:

What I really want is for you to intervene in this issue to ensure the best interests of women and their partners and families are served. There is a solution out there that is agreeable to women and staff if we all show flexibility and creativity, and there is real dialogue between ALL stakeholders, not just staff. My ultimate aim is to ensure that no woman is separated from her partner/support network when she receives bad news or has to make difficult decisions about her baby. And the recognition that a woman's partner or birth partner is not a visitor or an optional extra in maternity care, but an essential co-parent of the baby. I do not think this is an unreasonable thing to ask for, do you? And given the technologies we have available, every woman and her chosen partner should be able to fulfil their right to a family life.

If you can take the above forward in a positive manner, putting actions in place to remedy the issues raised above and taking us with you as joint stakeholders in our care, then I am not all that bothered about a formal response to this letter. However, in any response to this letter, please answer point by point and do not patronise or insult us by avoiding giving answers or by giving us silly answers to our serious questions. For this to work out for everyone, including the Trust, we need genuine and positive discussions and problem solving.

Looking forward to your commitment to sorting this out!

Every good wish
Ruth Weston

cc.

8 plus MPs; Leeds Councillor for Health and Wellbeing and Adults; Chair of scrutiny board (children and families); Leeds Council; Councillor Executive Member for Children and Families in Leeds; Baroness Julia Cumberlege; Matt Hancock, MP and Minister for Health; Professor Jacqueline Dunkley-Bent; BBC Radio 4, You and Yours

programme; National Childbirth Trust; Chair of Association for Improvement in Maternity Services; Maria Booker of Birthrights; Editor of *The Yorkshire Post.*

As you can see, it is polite but pulls no punches. Notice how I put the strong personal testimony at the top of the letter to ensure it was read first, as for many, this might be the only section that would be read. Also key to success was that the letter was copied to EVERYONE starting with Baroness Cumberlege, writer of the Better Births Report[27] and then Chair of the NHS England Maternity Transformation Stakeholder Council, through to the CEO/ Chairs of various national organisations, including lawyers, the 10 Leeds MPs, local CCG leads, and all the local media contacts I could find. In addition, I also published the letter on Twitter and tweeted on the subject for days.

There was a long silence from the Trust, but I chased a response up after a week using the lovely acknowledgement from Baroness Cumberlege to point out that it was not only a stroppy woman (i.e. me!) who was waiting for their response to my letter. I received an expected organisational response from the Trust that said nothing much in a lot of words. What did happen was that an announcement was made stating that partners could now attend most scans – and all the significant ones. Despite the initial messaging on the subject, it was clear that the sonographers are more fearful of video links to partners ending up in a court of law than catching Covid-19 from the two people in the room for a scan.

It was a win! And I had the name and contact of a senior staff member who said I could contact him . . .

Epilogue

This exchange of letters ran into the sand but the issue I had raised in my letter was by now a national debate, in newspapers, in Parliament and all over Twitter. Of course, Leeds, along with other Hospital Trusts, were now in the spotlight. The sonographer associations were also in the media defending their position and interestingly insulting the women and organisations that challenged them – always a sign that the opponent recognises the weakness of their own argument. Nevertheless, my life had thrown me a curveball, and this one-woman guerrilla attack was at an end: she disappeared into the undergrowth once more.

The Moral of This Tale:

- Take time to write a really good, clear letter – then send it to EVERYONE.

- Make sure your key points are clear and concise and highlight your solution to the issue, making sure that what you want them to do is doable.

- Do your research – it will be worth it.

- You do not always know the outcome of your letter, and some of the responses/outcomes (such as a note from Baroness Cumberlege) are not what you had looked for.

- Sometimes, as in this case, although they defend their position in writing, they will quietly change the policy to reduce the uncomfortable attention and heat.

- Sometimes, as in this case, the Trust is not the key problem: it was the sonographers who were refusing point blank to allow any recording of their sessions. The Trust were caught in the middle and clearly felt they did not have the leverage locally or nationally to force a change in the national Sonographer Association's policy on the matter.

- This whole episode shows how weak the leverage and power is of women and patients within the NHS. We don't have truly patient-centred care when patients do not have a seat at any negotiating table or significant leverage over difficult decisions.

- If you take action like this, you have done something significant and important, even if you have to give up because you have no more capacity. Be proud of yourself.

- It takes tenacity and a certain amount of bloody mindedness to do this sort of thing – and sometimes nerves of steel. So good luck with your letter!

Petitions

Petitions are another standard tool in the kit bag of a campaigner. Loved by some, hated by others, they can be like Marmite® amongst those seeking change. However, there is no doubt a petition can be an effective lever at local and national levels. My best successes with petitions were at a local level.

Calderdale Birth Centre Petition

The petition was a massive success from a campaigning point of view, but the spade work for success was done by the wonderful Lucy who worked for us at the time. Calderdale Birth Centre had closed for six weeks due to "staffing issues". For anyone with experience of birth centre closures, or anyone who has read Deborah Hughes' work (with M Kirkham and R Deery)[28], this was a red flag because "temporary closures" often lead to permanent ones.

Calderdale Birth Centre had been a flagship for birth centres in the area, was hugely popular with women in Bradford until they had their own birth centre, and had water births before any other local Trust – not to mention being a lovely place to have a baby. Rumour had it that so many women in Bradford chose to birth at Calderdale that it caused a financial row – indeed, this was one of the many arguments we threw at the Trust for our own birth centre.

And here it was being closed for 'staffing reasons'. This is generally organisation-speak for "We are running the place down and are pulling women and staff into the labour ward with a view to closing the birth centre in a couple of years due to lack of use and 'staffing issues'."

It is a regular tactic of Trusts wanting to close their birth centres (it was used by Shrewsbury and Telford Hospital Trust to close their rural MLUs, for instance), to pull midwives from the birth centre on a regular basis, closing the unit so often that mothers cannot make a real choice to go there, so numbers plummet. The unit is then closed permanently because it is "no longer financially viable" because mothers are not choosing to go there and "staffing issues". Any independent observer can see that the whole thing has been choreographed by the Trust concerned.

This was what I saw in the significant "temporary" closure of this pioneering unit. I checked the official hospital website and local media, and the same bland phrases without any commitment to the future opening of the MLU rang alarm bells.

I started to grumble and possibly rant about the situation in the office each day, and so it was that on Thursday when Lucy was in the office, she responded (after some time), "So why don't we set up a petition?"

She had called my bluff – why not do something instead of grumbling about it? Lucy set to work: a petition was set up that day with some careful wording and then follow-up campaign articles were created to go in a blog, in the Choices mailing, and Facebook posts.

I remember reading one of the promotional articles and blanching at its forthrightness in public.

"Maybe we tone it down," I suggested. "Where did you get the information?"

"You! I took notes of everything you have said and just wrote it up!" she replied.

I reflected. It was what I had said, although phrased for the privacy of my office rather than for public consumption! But then again, it was true! It was my opinion that this was the beginning of the end for the birth centre if we did not take action here and now.

So with some careful edits, it went out and I put on my hard hat and waited for the reaction. I also made a mental note to be more careful about what I said out loud in the office… that said, I had made that mental note before and ignored it!

The reaction took me by surprise; I watched, mesmerised, as the number of signatures grew exponentially and the shares on our postings increased.

Early in the following week, when I received a call from the Head of Midwifery, the signatures were well over a thousand and still growing. The RCM was involved at national level and figures in national maternity organisations were interested and contacting both me and the Head of Midwifery.

One of the really canny ideas I had was to look at my contacts book and start contacting the national leaders who I thought might be most influential in this situation. After a sticky start (I was a bit too 'Yorkshire direct'!), it was how I linked up personally with the wonderful Mary Newburn, one of the authors of the Birthplace Survey. She provided me with excellent advice on wording and strategy (frankly, making it much less inflammatory), pulled in some other heavy weights, and generally provided support.

The Head of Midwifery was clearly very angry when she rang me late one afternoon. I did not blame her at all; what had been a quiet, low-key temporary closure of a birth centre had become not only a local scandal, but was also becoming a national one. Possibly worst of all for a Head of Midwifery, it was causing reputational damage with her colleagues in the RCM and NHS England, which is a huge deal. The conversation was two hours long, and at the end of the conversation, she accepted that there had been a gross lack of communication with women and the public about the nature of the closure. In turn, I accepted her word that this was indeed a temporary closure due to genuine short-term staffing issues and that they had done their utmost to make a mini birth centre on the labour ward.

Where we probably disagreed was over the long-term policy for the unit. I wanted the default for low-risk women, who did not express a preference, to be the birth centre as it is the safest place for them to birth. She wanted it to remain an active choice for women to choose the birth centre. I saw this as an issue because it depended too much on the pro-birth centre support of maternity leaders and the provision of high-quality and timely information for mothers from their carers. Notably, there was an MSLC but it had faded away, primarily I think because the HOM found it a nuisance having an active forum for opinions contrary to hers. But in our conversation, she acknowledged the importance of it, because listening to those very women and professionals and discussing the closure with them may well have averted the very public row that had now occurred.

This is a recurring theme through all the major rows I have been involved in. If maternity leaders listened systematically to parents and their representatives and took their concerns seriously, they would avoid some major and public embarrassments. "Know thine enemy and keep them close" would be my motto for hospital managers! Keep your enemies in plain sight!

Neighbourhood Midwives

By contrast, another petition I set up failed miserably and it is useful to share the story to learn from it, as I did. When the effective, well-run independent midwifery practice, Neighbourhood Midwives (NM), had to pull out of their one NHS contract to provide continuity of carer to women because it was financially unviable, I, along with many others across the country, was furious. One to One Midwives had also gone out of business for the same reasons, demonstrating that for all the rhetoric of delivering continuity of carer and all the noise about enabling independent practice to contract into the NHS (much like GP surgeries), the system had stacked the odds against midwives practising autonomously within the NHS (though notably not obstetricians…) and delivering real continuity of midwifery carer with all its benefits.

Someone else quickly put up a petition decrying what had happened and, expressing support, signatures quickly gathered pace as people reacted with sadness, love and outrage at what had happened. However, suddenly the petition was closed saying "Victory!" But there had been no victory at all! We learnt that NM leaders had asked for the petition to be taken down because the wording had not been appropriate. They wanted to thank everyone for the support but although change was needed, a simple reinstatement of the contract was not.

I was upset. I felt that the person who started the petition could have discussed and negotiated better wording for the petition with NM leaders. I felt that there was a bigger picture that could have been worked with, taking the heat away from them whilst using their situation as an example of what needed to change in maternity. And most certainly there are many ways to close a petition, but calling something a 'victory' where there is patently none is not one of them! I think it may have been inexperience on the part of the petitioner and it was sad, because a team of us working together could have used such good will and support for NM to leverage change, or at least some accountability.

I decided to see if I could relaunch a petition along these lines and laboured many hours with a friend to get the wording and tone right. I launched, pushed it and blogged it but it got nowhere; the impetus had gone. The chance lost.

The Moral of This Tale:

- A petition can work very well as a strategic tool to bring opponents to the negotiating table, publicise your cause and draw together a campaign team for further action. Do not expect more from a petition than this.

- Timing can be crucial for the success of a petition.

- A petition can also test the public appetite for your issue at this time. This is important: if you have put up a good petition and it has gone nowhere, then evaluate and learn. It may well be the wrong tool for this cause at this particular time.

- It works best as a team effort – although this should not stop you from setting up a petition on your own if that is the only option.

- Pool resources and take criticism generously. Be prepared to change the wording of the petition and even the tone, as more information becomes available and wise heads advise. What you want is a petition that is effective in reaching your goal, so swallow your pride. With the successful birth centre petition, we amended wording for clarity and accuracy when both friends and opponents messaged us. For instance, I remember Mary Newburn commenting on my use of the Birthplace Cohort Study, "This is really powerful evidence in your favour so you don't need to overstate it." Good advice. I changed the wording.

Chapter 7

❧

Media Skills for the Campaigner

SOCIAL MEDIA IS ONE thing but getting involved with the general media is another, and for me it was a daunting prospect at the beginning. However, it is something we have to tackle because the only way most ordinary folk can get a hearing or hold an institution to account, is to threaten or cause actual public embarrassment and reputational damage.

Here is an overview of my journey and the important skills I learnt along the way. Remember, these are not the words of a professional lobbyist or public relations professional, but my advice as a jobbing grassroots campaigner for other jobbing grassroots campaigners.

The Local Newspaper et al.

My first attempts at getting stories into the local press were quite tentative. I was a chaplain to students at the time and I wanted to get stories in the local paper about student poverty and poor student housing. I learnt how to write a press release and that to raise an issue, you **have** to tell a story – there has to be a human face to an issue you want to discuss.

Five Important Things To Know if You Want To Get an Item in the Local or National Press:

- You need a compelling, even outrageous, title that will attract or hook a bored journalist.

- You need to ensure that you encapsulate your story in the first couple of sentences. This may be all that anyone will read, so make sure it packs a punch. *Then* you can go into more detail, retelling the story at a slower pace. If you read articles in local newspapers, this is how they are structured.

- You need to have a human interest. Whether it is you or someone else, there has to be a story to gain the interest of the reader.

- If you want to ensure printing, then a photograph is a must. Maternity, of course, is an easy sell as mothers and babies are so photogenic! I have had articles published without sending a photograph with the press release, but this has usually been because they liked the story so much, they sent their own photographer or found a stock photo from their archive.

- Try to have a couple of quotes in your press release. This can be from the person who is the human interest and from a local 'expert' or 'campaigner'. Of course, you can quote yourself in any of these roles.

I really got a handle on getting into the local press and media when I took over Aquabirths. I had no money and, with four little ones, no time, so I set myself the target of featuring in the local newspaper every two months for whatever reason! Of course, the first story was about a mother pregnant with her fourth child buying the company because she wanted a water birth. For a while, the local reporters called me the 'Remington Woman' from the old TV advert ("I liked it so much, I bought the company!"). I was prepared to get in my swimming cozzy and fill the birth pool for a photo session with me and the kids, so I had a whole page article on page 3. You must understand that you have to be dead to get on the front page (!), then there was national news on page 2 – so page 3 is the place to be. The photo of me in the pool was recycled for so many other articles! I was on the business pages (near the back before the sport!), in articles on family life, the budget, growing your own, etc., etc., etc. I did not care, so long as I had that line "Local businesswoman and mother, Ruth Weston…" This was pre-social media and I was simply wanting to ensure people knew that me and my pools existed.

There are two other important points that are still relevant to campaigning today, even with the power and reach of social media as a campaign tool:

- People have said to me that no one reads local papers anymore. That may or may not be true but I know for sure that local politicians (and service providers) read the local papers and they REALLY don't like an article or story that trashes their policy, reputation or service. Even the threat of being in the local paper can bring some people to the negotiating table.

- However, there can be some close relationships between the editorial team and, for instance, your local hospital, which will keep your fabulous story out. Here is an example of what happened to me.

The Tale of the Disappearing Tale!

It was announced that the local Trust was going to get rid of the Early Pregnancy Assessment Unit (EPAU) at Bradford Royal Infirmary. I was horrified. As you know from my story, my first miscarriage was managed on a large general gynaecological ward alongside booked terminations, and much else. It was not a good experience. The small specialist EPAU had still been a trial for me after my previous trauma, but with its small ward rooms, kind specialist staff and its own sonography room where women could see their baby on screen, it was a much kinder and gentler place to absorb difficult news.

I rang the health correspondent at the local paper – by this time, I knew the team well – and told her how upset I was about this decision. I gave her my story of what it was like having a miscarriage on a general gynae ward. I knew it was a good story – the sort of story that could land on page 3. She was hooked, as I knew she would be, and said she would certainly get back to me. Then… radio silence.

After a few days, I got back to her to see what was happening about my story. There were some awkward pauses and careful wording – one of those conversations where everything had to be in code because it was more than their job's worth. My understanding of the conversation is that she was running with the story but it was 'sat on' from on high. The chief editor was known to be close to key city leaders and I suspect the story was stopped. That said, so was the closure of the EPAU, so maybe my story did the trick without being published!

My experience was that most negative health stories would not get published in our local newspaper. And certainly my questions at the AGM – however entertaining and newsworthy – did not get in the paper either, when other (less entertaining) questions did. If I wanted to have an issue raised, I learnt it needed a positive spin for the hospital or to be a feature providing information with some references to negative experiences. We therefore sought out other places to place our negative campaigning health stories. They did not appear in our local paper.

The Moral of This Tale:

- **As with working with allies (see Chapter 8), you may have to swallow your pride and anger and change the tone and style of your story in order to have it published.**

- It may be unfair that the press is not as independent as you feel it should be, but you are not calling the shots here. Find out or work out how you need to present your story to get it published and use that knowledge to get published.

- Make allies of reporters and correspondents. They will guide you, even if sometimes it is coded and implied.

- Remember, you can try elsewhere with the uncut version of your story as well.

- Finally, remember that as a campaigner, sometimes the story does not have to be published to get the desired result.

Radio and TV Tactics

Radio and TV were even more daunting for this fledgling campaigner back in the day. My employer kindly enabled me to join a twilight media training workshop for voluntary groups early on in my chaplaincy student poverty campaign. I took the training on radio and TV interviews to heart, especially as I heard politicians using these very tactics every day on the news. We practised interviewing each other, which came in really handy in my first radio interview a few days later.

I share the top tips I learnt for interviews for your benefit:

- Prepare for the interview. Make sure you know your topic well and have the facts at your fingertips. And certainly make sure that you know more than your interviewer!

- Decide what your message is going to be to your audience – rehearse it so you can sum it up in a pithy sentence or two. This is the message you want to get across in the interview and weave into every answer, no matter what they ask!

- Think about the questions you may be asked. Have three points you want to make about your message, in answer to these questions.

- Be prepared for the question with a catch or twist designed to take you off balance and off message – and there is usually one, especially if they perceive you to be a seasoned campaigner. When it happens, sometimes you can come out with a brilliant riposte, but if not, give yourself a chance to think of an answer, breathe, count, ask the interviewer to repeat the question, remember your message, and go for it.

- Keep answers concise and try not to waffle.

- Interviewing improves with practice and skill. Do not take it personally if things go wrong, especially if it is a difficult interview. There are many reasons why this happened, so evaluate it, learn from it, move on. Do not take it personally.

A Hypothetical Interview Preparation

I am being called to interview on the Save Independent Midwifery campaign.

My message: As families, we are wanting to save independent midwifery to ensure we can continue to choose the kind of safe care we want, and have the kinds of births we want.

Three points:

1. Medical evidence from *The Lancet* papers shows that having a midwife you know and trust reduces premature birth, stillbirth and miscarriage by around 20%. It reduces pain and interventions and reduces postnatal depression. If the only way to have this care is to employ an independent midwife, what is there not to love?

2. Having an independent midwife is extremely costly for some families, but the cost of poor care and poor outcomes at birth and postnatally is far more expensive in the long run. Surely a healthy happy mother and baby is priceless and we should as a country invest in that?

3. Independent midwifery is not being banned because it is unsafe – their outcomes are second to none – but because the rules for insurance are changing. It is a complex area, but solutions can and should be found so women can choose this safe form of care if they want it.

Possible Trick Questions

- Something around private health care is for rich people.

- Isn't independent midwifery being banned because it is unsafe?

Here is how the hypothetical interview works out:

First question: *Independent midwifery is for rich people who can afford to pay, isn't it?* (Trick question first, which is very naughty!)

My answer: Families are choosing independent midwifery because this is the only way we can get the kind of safe care we want and the birth we want. Medical evidence shows that continuity of midwifery carer reduces stillbirth, miscarriage, premature birth and interventions such as forceps and C-sections. Surely this is what everyone wants? For my last child, we spent *all* our savings on an independent midwife because we decided a good birth with a healthy mother and baby are priceless.

Second question: *So, tell me why have you set up the Saving Independent Midwifery Facebook campaign*

My answer: I set up the Facebook group on a whim because I was afraid that me and my friends would not be able to get the kind of safe care and birth we wanted on the NHS and then be unable to choose it via an independent midwife. I thought it would just be a few friends in Yorkshire who would join! But it turned into a massive national campaign, showing how important it is to lots of families that they can get the kind of care that only independent midwives currently guarantee. Lots of midwives have joined because this is not about competition; it is about upholding high standards of maternity care here in the UK.

<u>Third question.</u> *Why is independent midwifery threatened?*

<u>My answer:</u> Independent midwifery is not being banned because it is unsafe – their outcomes and safety are second to none – but because the rules for insurance are changing. It is a complex area because insurance in maternity does not work like insurance in the normal world. But solutions can be found, and should be found, because the data shows that it is safe care with very good outcomes, even for high-risk pregnancies, and women and families want it. Surely the country wants the best for its mothers and babies – so why not invest in it?

Conclusion

For the introverts amongst us, the thought of a televised interview will make you sick. For me, I loved interviews; I loved the cut and thrust and wing and a prayer of live interviews. If you like interviews, go for it! If you don't, make sure that if you get landed with one, you know the basics so you can get by.

Lady Luck: Getting on TV and Radio

It is all very well being worried about the interview, but first they must want to talk to you! Getting your story on radio and television is a matter of knowing the right people or having the right contacts, approaching them at the right time in terms of that week's news agenda, being willing to drop everything to go to a studio or for them to come to you, and, of course, you need luck.

As an ordinary campaigner, there is no magic bullet for getting your story in front of the news agenda.

Radio Leeds called me up regularly because I got on to their database, sometimes as an expert businesswoman talking about birth, breastfeeding and family matters, and sometimes as a Bradford Mum with five kids.

Airedale Mums were featured on *Look North* (BBC local news programme) because the presenter had recently had a baby and their story resonated with her – and she had a personal connection to the group too. Airedale Mums pooled their skills, parenting and connections to speak on local radio stations and get into the local newspapers too. These photogenic, techno-savvy articulate mums used their skills to highlight what all women and birthing people want – good care, respect and a real choice about where and how they birth. In the end, the hospital had to begin dealing with these women and their legitimate concerns, because their failure to do so was resulting in poor media coverage. As Chair of the MSLC, it gave me the leverage alongside progressive NHS managers, in arguing for proper home birth cover, support for water birth, midwifery-led units (birth centres), and respect and support for what clinicians started calling "unusual choices" rather than the previous "refusing medical advice".

I was interviewed for Radio 4's PM programme, and featured on the BBC News at Six in the same week because some weeks earlier, I had posted a comment (and a brief outline of my story) on the BBC website after a programme about birth on Radio 4. The programme was talking about the history of birth in the UK and I was so incensed by the programme, I let chaos reign in the house whilst I wrote on their contact form that the attitudes and care talked about on the programme were still prevalent today and happening to me of all people.

I did not expect any response because it had not happened before. I forgot about it until a few weeks later, my husband rang up as I drove back from a meeting at Airedale Hospital, to say the BBC had been trying to get in touch with me! They had a news item and wanted a human-interest story to be part of it. Two big BBC vans with satellite dishes appeared in our little cul-de-sac. The whole family sat in line, in order of age, including my husband (!), with me at the end of the line speaking to a vase on the mantelpiece (!). This was because the shot needed to look like I was talking to someone across the room and not to camera. Yes, it felt weird! I said my piece (whilst being courteous, of course), and perhaps it is the only time I truly felt I was able to express the importance of good maternity care to a big audience that might change political agendas. I even have my own BBC website page, complete with a lovely photo of me and baby no. 5 at the beach together.[29]

I was featured in the TV series *Desperate Midwives* because I was the only current client of my independent midwife who was bonkers enough to be willing to have a camera following me around. This gave me space to talk in-depth about the important benefits of having a midwife you know and trust, and demonstrate those benefits with my story. My good home birth with laughter and loving support, ending with being tucked up in bed with a sleeping husband and happy baby was in sad contrast to the experience of most of the women in the documentary. Having a midwife or two that you know and trust throughout the maternal pathway makes a massive difference to outcomes: and here it was, demonstrated in my own life, in my own pool, in glorious technicolour. You can still find me forever giving birth if you Google it!

I spotted and responded to a call for participants, which resulted in a fun few weeks featuring on an afternoon programme called *Cash for Trash*, where I sold all my junk and gave half the proceeds to a chosen charity (AIMS, of course!), which gave me a lovely slot to describe the important work AIMS does.

And so it went on. I took opportunities wherever I found them, and so, for that matter, did Airedale Mums. We were passionate about our message, we had lovely children, and we were full of fun as well as passion.

The Moral of This Tale:

- **If you want to have your say in the general media, use all your contacts, and be shameless in seeking out any and every opportunity to get behind a mic, in front of a camera or to have your words in print.**

- **Most (although not all) TV and radio programmes are not the place for the hard words of letters and meetings; they are somewhere to use wit and human stories to highlight what a difference** decent maternity care makes to the lives of mothers and their families. Of course, it does concentrate minds if an email from the person they have just seen or heard on TV or radio drops into their inbox...

- If they like your style, researchers will return to you again and again for another entertaining story, a pithy point and a good photo.

- Finally, don't think it is a waste of time to type a response or some feedback to a radio or TV episode or to drop a line to the editor of a paper – it often leads to nothing but there is always that one day when you get a phone call... may Lady Luck go with you!

Social Media

In no way am I going to teach social media to the digital natives coming after me, so some hard-won learning points and a story will suffice.

- **Never ever** write anything on social media that you don't want the whole world to know forever. Treat it like a microphone – assume it is always live.

- It is important to grasp that your personal self and your campaigning self on social media are very different people. Social media has an unhappy knack of entangling these two, causing difficulty and hurt as a result. Even if social media entwine these personas, you must be clear about the boundaries between the two, and guard your privacy and personal relationships accordingly.

- Be careful what you say and how you say it, especially in social media groups – particularly those throwaway remarks that slip out when you might be tired or stressed. What you might think you are saying, and how you may think you are saying it, may not be read as such by someone else. We all come to our human interactions with filters and vulnerabilities from past exchanges with others. It is so easy to misread what someone else means, or for someone to misread what you have said; and it is then so easy for a row to ensue based on these misunderstandings, assumptions and vulnerabilities. A row that may result in a broken relationship. I have too often been saddened when two or three fantastic women have a row based on a misunderstanding, which ends relationships and weakens the strong campaign groups they are part of. To this day, I regret a throwaway remark I made on a Facebook group when I was tired and ill; it was misunderstood by a journalist and ended a media relationship. These sorts of things are so easily done and so hard to undo, so please be aware, and beware of everything you say on social media, especially in your campaigning role.

- Be swift to apologise, edit or delete even if the remark was not meant the way it was taken. Relationships are more important than a message on a chat group.

- My motto for all interactions is to **be kind**. You can be tough and kind, you can 'tell truth to power' and be kind, you can challenge and be kind, you can be angry and be kind. It is holding the person or organisation with the same respect and regard as you would want for yourself – simply that – because one day we may need correcting and we would want the same space to apologise, edit or delete. This also means that if someone misunderstands and reacts strongly to your posting, you don't react, and certainly not immediately. Let things calm down, let people cool off, and allow them space to retract, delete or apologise – or plain ignore it if you can.

- For some of us, speaking the truth on social media can result in an outpouring or avalanche of vitriol and abuse. I hurt for you – I do. This is really tough. As with any situation of conflict (see Chapter 9), breathe, keep steady, keep focused, don't react right away, look for what is going on behind the smoke and the noise, and then plan how to respond to that. Seek support and help where you need it. Some people have friends or allies who edit and delete the horrible stuff from their social media so they don't have to read it all. Step back if you need to. Your life and well-being are worth more than this! Finally, if you see it happening to someone else, know how important it is to show support for the person, whilst not adding to the conflict.

- **Never** insult anyone on social media (it is not kind and it does not work) and **never** trade personal insults because that does not work either! Actually, don't do it in real life either! It is not courteous, it is not kind, it is not professional, it does not build allies and it does not resolve issues, so it is of no tactical use at all. Indeed, a good opponent will see this as a weakness, as I would (see Chapter 9), and will play it to their advantage.

- Sometimes you will post stuff and there is little reaction – indeed, sometimes you post stuff for months with little reaction – and then one day it takes off and you are suddenly in the middle of a media whirlwind! The same advice applies as in a conflict situation: keep steady, keep focused, don't react right away, look for what is really going on behind the smoke and noise, and carefully plan your next move accordingly to get the best out of this opportunity.

Saving Independent Midwifery: Lessons Learnt From a Campaign Facebook Group

It was February 2018 and independent midwifery was under threat again. I was in bed ill with a virus, it was a few months after my first physical breakdown, and a few months before I started my long sabbatical to recover from my mental and emotional burnout. I was well enough to be bored in bed and incensed enough at what I was reading on Facebook to do something about it, so decided to set up a campaign Facebook group. I still had a strong network in Yorkshire and I felt sure we could get together to support our Yorkshire independent midwives. I set up a 'Saving Independent Midwifery in Yorkshire' group, invited key network contacts, thinking that as in the past, a group of 6 to 30 of us could collectively organise letter writing, lobbying MPs, petitions and various campaign-type stuff. How wrong I was! In a few days, there were hundreds of us.

Then an independent midwife – God bless her as the amazing campaigner and midwife she is – rang me and said she had seen my group, but to have the impact, it needed more members and she was going to sort it. And she did. Whilst driving about the countryside between appointments, she rang up every contact she had (and she had a lot!) and invited them to join the group. In a few days, we had 2,000 members and growing. I had changed the group's name to 'Saving Independent Midwifery' – as the reach was clearly way beyond Yorkshire!

Learning Points

I had never run a Facebook group of this size and the learning curve was steep. Here are my learning points:

- It was quickly very clear that some 'rules of engagement' on the group were going to be necessary. The 'nice' me thinks that everyone knows you should not trade personal insults and that you should always post with respect and courtesy, but in the real world, it is necessary to pin these rules at the top of the group to make sure everyone is clear how things MUST be.

- Then, of course, you have to enforce them, and enforce them rigorously. 'Nice' me did not like doing this, so I would message people privately appealing to their better selves, or I would post into discussions requests to keep to the issue rather than personal argument. On a smaller, more intimate groups, this might work, but on this megalith of a group, the instruments had to be harder and blunter.

- There is no way anyone can moderate a group of that size on their own because people are posting literally 24/7; bear in mind it was a group of parents and midwives so included night feeders and healthcare professionals going on and off shift! I picked half a dozen moderators I believed I could trust, who were level-headed, and who spanned the professional and participant spectrum.

- Good cop/bad cop. I am kind; I want to give everyone the benefit of the doubt and give people time and space to work things out. In a big group, there is neither the time nor the relationship to do this. One of the moderators I recruited had moderated large public groups before; she was a straight-talking Texan and she would take no shit. There was plenty of it flying about in the first few weeks, with misunderstandings, vulnerabilities, taking offence, insults, etc. She set up the group to stream on her screen whilst she was working so she could quickly pick up a discussion turning nasty. She acted right away, warning participants, blocking postings and throwing people off the group if they did not comply. I blanched at how tough she was! Some people I respect took offence to her tough stance on compliance to the rules (which were, after all, about tolerance and respect!), and frankly, I found it uncomfortable at times. But it has to be said that after a couple of weeks, the group settled down, the 'bunfights', as she called them, stopped, providing more space for constructive discussion and action. Maybe a gentler touch could have worked; some people certainly thought this to be the case, and I do not say they are wrong.

- However, for a large campaign group to be effective, for every participant to be respected and listened to, we have to ensure that rules of courtesy and tolerance are adhered to, without exception. There is no easy way to do this, especially in a very large, fast-paced group.

The Impact

The internal workings of the group are one thing, but the group was also having an impact externally. Hundreds of parents and midwives were writing to their MP, to the Government Minister for Health, to the NHS England Chief Executive, to the NHS England Head of Midwifery, and others. In addition, hundreds of people contacted the Nursing and Midwifery Council who were, via their interpretation and enforcement, pushing independent midwifery and the mothers' choice of this care to extinction. If their existence was to protect the public interest, then we thought their actions showed they were not fit for purpose.

A few weeks after the launch of the group, I found myself in a room at the RCM headquarters in London, discussing the future autonomy and health of professional midwifery with key national figures. We also discussed strategies to improve the future prospects of midwifery and independent midwifery in the UK. What put me there was being the founder of the Saving Independent Midwifery Facebook group, and I knew it.

At one point, I said to Cathy Warwick, then CEO of the RCM, and someone I respected immensely, "If it feels we are being uncomfortably loud and forceful putting pressure on you to act, this is not meant as personal criticism to you or the RCM. Our strategy is to give you the cover and the leverage to go into your meetings with the NMC and say things have to change – because here is evidence of the strong public and professional outcry at your current policy and actions."

Essentially, we, the campaigners, were playing bad cop to the RCM good cop. She understood it and so thankfully our relationship remained good across the divide.

It was also because of the Facebook group that I had a place in a meeting with the then CEO of the NMC. I pressed her (she was a lawyer rather than a clinician, and a policy head rather than a parent) on how she knew she was acting in the public interest, as she maintained she was, when she had to admit they did not actually have any interaction with the interested public – parents and families or the organisations that represent them. I still find it astonishing that the NMC was enforcing policy on midwifery and maternity without ANY engagement with organisations such as the NCT, AIMS, Doula UK and the many other parenting organisations that could inform them of what the public interest in maternity means in real life. I doubt anything much has changed here, and it makes me so angry that decisions that affect our births and well-being 'in our interests' are made by people that don't think we are important enough to consult, let alone have a seat at the decision-making table!

As with many such campaign movements, it slowly faded as the energy dissipated and we had to put energy into the lives and jobs of our everyday worlds. As a leader, I had a key part in that: I had to step back as my health once again began to deteriorate. My withdrawal was so entire that I was unaware when the battle for independent midwifery in the UK was lost. Will my daughters have the choice of a highly skilled professional midwife who is independent of the NHS's patriarchal systems at their births? I don't know and that grieves me greatly. I wish so much I could have fought on.

The Moral of This Tale:

- **Facebook is one of many social media platforms and may well not be the premier one for campaigning as you read this book. BUT the principles still apply, that one day a post may go viral or a group you set up suddenly experiences exponential and sudden growth and it is difficult to keep up.**

- **Learn the lessons shared here and from other people with experience, because these opportunities can have a massive positive impact if handled well.**

- **Also keep your eyes open for any new social media platforms that may be more effective for your campaign. Good luck and good campaigning!**

Chapter 8

❧

Finding Your Allies

SUCCESS NEEDS ALLIES. Allies are the people who work with you, or deliberately choose not to stand in your way, in making change happen. These people can be your friends and family, they can be people who gather around a single issue or a similar set of experiences, they can be professionals who agree with you and want to seek change, they can be politicians, journalists, senior managers and leaders, or even, on occasion, your opponents. To be successful in campaigning, you need to be adept at seeking them out and cultivating them. The wider the spectrum of your allies, the harder it is for your opposition to legitimise itself, the more sides you have from which to attack, and the larger the pool for effective ideas and strategies. Sometimes you can turn opponents into allies to, for instance, gain a birth centre, and this is a real win. Here are some thoughts and experiences around finding and working with your allies.

Finding Your Allies: Airedale Mums

Looking back, I have never been quite sure how it began: the small conversations that set things in motion were not recognised as significant until afterwards. Me and a local independent midwife, independently of each other, were chatting to our clients who were upset with the care they had received from the local Airedale NHS Trust, and put them in touch with others with whom we had had a similar conversation. I don't know what we thought might happen – maybe we expected mutual friendship and support, maybe mutual encouragement when making a complaint. What actually happened was all their own work. Extraordinary, and a tribute to these mothers who went way beyond the call of duty. It shows how a dozen intelligent tech- and media-savvy women can disrupt the culture of maternity services and make space for something better.

What They Did:

- They attended MSLC meetings as a group of mums with their babies and toddlers, often discomforting the commissioners with their lack of facility and accommodation for parents. They asked questions, raised issues and generally made the MSLC work for mums. Coming together as a group gave them the strength to ensure their voice was heard: they made themselves very difficult to ignore. I absolutely loved the meetings when they brought flapjacks and friends – filling the room with the hum of babies and toddlers, and changing the dynamic of every conversation.

- They wrote letters to the Head of Midwifery and successfully sought meetings to discuss their concerns and solutions to improve maternity care. They contacted local MPs and one MP agreed to meet them, listened to their stories and picked the issue up on their behalf.

- They used their network to contact local media and, as a result, appeared on local television news, local radio and newspapers. This caused a huge amount of consternation from the Trust concerned but it certainly forced the Trust to put their house in order in regard to home birth cover, and enabled me as Chair of MSLC to shift some policies and practices which were at issue.

- They put in Freedom of Information (FOI) Requests for information that the Trusts had refused to provide to the MSLC (although they should have done). As a result of taking this action, not only could we see the outcomes of their policies and practices (such as the number of closures, home births, C-sections, etc.) but also the Trusts 'gave in' and started providing the information voluntarily, because it was obvious that they were going to start getting monthly FOI Requests if they did not!

- The Airedale Mums made an excellent and detailed formal complaint to Monitor (supposedly an organisation to hold commissioners and providers to the rules and standards) about the behaviour of the health commissioning body towards an independent midwifery practice (One to One Midwives) operating in the area providing gold standard care to tariff. However, the response that eventually came back stated that although the rules had been broken, Monitor were not going to take action. So much for accountability and putting the well-being of mothers first!

- Every single one of the mums took on training and qualifications which enabled them to support other mothers and parents, some taking highly responsible and professional roles within organisations that support families and midwives.

This group of mums had an impact far beyond their numbers, and because of their commitment and enthusiasm, continue to influence care and support mothers today. I cannot speak too highly of these women. Working with and alongside Airedale Mums was a joy and a pleasure!

The Moral of This Tale:

- **NEVER underestimate the impact you personally can have as a determined person doing what you can, when you can.**

- **NEVER underestimate the power and impact that a small group of determined mums and/or dads, techno-savvy and media friendly, can have on a maternity system.**

- **NEVER underestimate the impact of putting people who share an issue or a problem in touch with each other. Nor the role of supporting, encouraging or facilitating a group of parents,** midwives, students, etc. to do something effective about their concerns.

- Banding together as a group, combining strengths, skills and knowledge, childcare and personal contacts – the sum is greater than the individuals concerned. And it is far more sustainable, far more effective and far more fun working together – if nothing else, there is always someone else up at 2 am feeding the baby and having a brilliant idea, reading a policy or writing a letter!

Finding Your Allies: Working With Philip Davies, MP

I found one of my best supporters and allies in the campaign for better maternity care in Bradford was an MP with a reputation at the time for being a right-wing Conservative, well-known for his support of men's rights campaign groups and his seat on the Equalities Parliamentary Group where he advocated on the rights of men. There was a colourful feminist group in his constituency that campaigned specifically against him, and the truth is that I would probably have joined their ranks if he wasn't also an ally!

What made him an ally?

Airedale Mums were wondering how to effectively raise their concerns to bring about changes in maternity care and attitudes. They decided to contact the recently elected MP for Shipley and Bingley Rural, Philip Davies, and asked him to meet them and listen to their concerns. He was both tactful and sensitive – something many feminists in Shipley would be amazed to hear. The first thing that impressed us was that he suggested he came to us rather than us coming to him. The most impressive thing, however, was that he listened with empathy and comprehended the situation beyond what he was told.

It was arranged that the MP met Airedale Mums at the home of one of the members with his wife, also a good and tactful move. There he found half a dozen women with at least one baby/toddler each. I was present too. Rather than beginning with the agenda of our concerns, the mums in turn told their stories, and out of that, the issues were obvious: being listened to; having views and decisions respected; providing timely and accurate information in an impartial and respectful way; enabling and allowing choice; provision of staffing for home births; and so on. The stories told the tale we wanted to tell and the MP heard it and, by his responses, understood the underlying implications.

From this day forward, he was the most effective highly-placed ally we had in the district. I would regularly email or visit him to brief him on what was happening in maternity and the concerns I had.

In turn, he asked Parliamentary Questions, sent FOIs, asked awkward questions at meetings with the Trust and health commissioning body executives, and gave me information, feedback and comment about what was going on. He faithfully forwarded letter after letter raising my concerns on maternity policy nationally and locally to the relevant ministers. He was a stalwart of the maternity campaign and

I valued his support immensely, and still do. Philip Davies listened to his constituents and then represented their views and concerns in places we could not go and to people we could not meet. I suspect he did it without necessarily agreeing with everything I or Airedale Mums said and did. That made him a first-class ally.

Thoughts About Working With an Ally Who Would Normally Be an Opponent

What interested me then and now was my approach to him on my regular visits. We were not natural political allies, but I think two things enabled us to work together: First, his empathy and understanding of the human stories the mothers told – with the ability to place them in the wider NHS policy and political context. Second, when I approached him about these issues, I thought about HIS interests, concerns and political viewpoint and presented mine in that context.

When talking about place of birth, continuity of midwifery carer and about saving independent midwifery, I presented it in terms of women's right to choose the care that is right for them, about women being able to choose the place of their birth and who cares for them. I talked about how, if the NHS is not willing or able to deliver continuity of midwifery carer throughout the maternal pathway, then midwifery practices, such as One to One Midwives and Yorkshire Storks, should be allowed and enabled to do so, contracted either by the NHS or directly by women. This played well with his politics but also provided him with the political arguments and language to take it forward.

The Moral of This Tale:

- What you need to fully understand is that although I agreed with everything I was saying to him, in my usual political arena I would have presented it differently. Indeed, if Philip had been a left-leaning Labour MP, I would have presented my case very differently indeed (and did).

- The thing about issues such as maternity, climate change, homelessness, social care and so on, is that these are not party-political issues and many, if not all, of the solutions are not party political either. In the end, it is the language and the pathways that differ. If we make these issues party political, we will be hostage to the fortunes of the political winds. What we want to do is make maternity care better, whichever way the political wind is blowing. This being the case, we need to build our allies as communities of interest across the spectrum, working with the interests and understandings of our different allies to enable them to work effectively for a shared goal. This can mean we work with people who in any other situation we might view as our opponent.

- MPs are meant to work on behalf of their constituents, whatever particular party they represent, so it is right to assume that they might be supportive if you persuaded them of your case. This is also true of other elected representatives, such as local councillors.

Finding Your Allies: Working Across Professional Boundaries and Being the Critical Friend

There is much to be gained by HCPs and families working together. Health goals otherwise unreachable can be met in cooperation, information otherwise unavailable to either side can be shared, and really understanding how the other side lives and thinks, can make the world of difference in discussing difficult or controversial topics. Mutual trust and respect gained in working relationships enable such discussions to happen. However, we must be clear for the benefit of some professionals and some parents that cooperation, trust and respect does **not** mean that professionals and parents have to agree with one another, do as they are told, or not disagree strongly and even publicly at certain points.

My role as lay-Chair of the MSLC meant I had to be impartial. Some Chairs understand this to mean you cannot speak up for mothers and families or elevate their voices because that breaks the impartiality rule. I see it very differently: in maternity services, women and birthing people have few, if any, opportunities to have their voices heard at strategic and managerial levels: the MSLC (now MNVP) is one of the few places.

In a setting where mothers, especially black and minority ethnic mothers, have so little say about the care they receive, making greater space for women and birthing people to speak, elevating or amplifying their voices, is not *breaking* impartiality but *enabling* impartiality – levelling the playing field of power and influence a little to ensure some kind of equality.

In addition, maternity is a service for mothers and their families; it needs to deliver healthy and happy mothers, babies and families, and needs to deliver excellent care. If it is not doing so in any way, then it is not breaking any impartiality rule to point this out and elevate the voices of mothers and their families to ensure they are heard. And that is what happened. On the other hand, in a cooperative environment, understanding the challenges professionals faced enabled us to harness my role to leverage change that professionals were unable to achieve by internal means alone.

"Ask the Question – Just Ask the Question"

It was coming up to some big conference, possibly the Trust's AGM. My habit in later years was to let it be known that if professionals needed a question asked, then they could approach me in confidence.

One of the senior maternity managers quietly approached me in person and said, "Can you ask a question?"

"Of course. What do you want me to ask?"

"Ask a question about the birth centre."

"What answer will I get?"

"Just ask the question."

And she disappeared.

Bradford is a large unit with 6,000 births and evidence shows that low-risk women do not fare well in an obstetric unit with only 57.6% of them having a physiological birth, as opposed to 76% for low-risk women birthing in an alongside birth centre or MLU.[30] And so we needed a birth centre in Bradford. One was promised, the funding had been agreed we thought, but then a big silence... So I asked the question. I don't remember the wording except that it was phrased as an assumption that the agreed birth centre would be built; it was a question of timing. As readers will now know, the question itself was not as important as watching the Trust management's reaction to the assumption that they were delivering the birth centre as promised. And the answer was a big silence filled in with a lot of meaningless words.

At the next MSLC meeting, the question of how to bring pressure to bear was discussed. The Commissioner, a regular opponent, suggested with a twinkle in her eye, "Maybe you should write one of your letters, Ruth!"

We all laughed because she had been on the receiving end a few times – but this is exactly what I did. And it worked. The senior managers of the Trust suddenly started talking to the maternity managers about releasing the funding for the promised birth centre.

Once again, a case of playing good cop, bad cop, but using the teamwork of parents and professionals to reach a shared goal for the benefit of mothers and babies.

The Moral of This Tale:

- The phrase "Ask the question – just ask the question", has rung in my ears ever since this incident. Ask the question and see where it takes you. Your question may provide leverage for a professional on the inside to gain traction to a mutual goal, or your loud voice may provide cover or protection to allow weaker voices in the organisation to speak up.

- What it also demonstrates is that opponents can become allies in certain situations, if there is mutual respect behind the tensions.

- Lastly, it demonstrates how parents and professionals can work together across boundaries to achieve shared goals unreachable on their own.

Working Across Professional Boundaries: The Quality of Leadership

Julie Walker was a brilliant Head of Midwifery. Rather than trying to freeze out women like me, labelled 'troublemakers' for calling out the poor care we received, she brought us in, listened to and respected us, and gave us a seat at the table where decisions could be made. By doing so, we stopped being troublemakers (mostly!) and became part of the solution to the issues we raised. After all, that is what most people want when they complain; they want to stop it happening to anyone else. Why does the NHS have so much trouble with that?

Julie called me 'her friend and thorn in her side', and I trusted and respected her completely. I still do, wherever she may now be. Because our relationship was built on trust, I was able to provide information in confidence that gave her notice of issues that could blow up, and I was able to gain another perspective from her to the one I knew. This mutual trust and teamwork meant we were able to head off trouble before it caused damage or mitigate the damage it was going to cause. One small example may suffice to show the quality of lead we had.

Early in her post as Head of Midwifery, Julie came to a Choices meeting. But she did not come with the big hat on; she came in unobtrusively, sat quietly out of the way, introduced herself simply as a midwife and just listened, not intervening at any point. This was significant because on this occasion, there was a discussion on gestational diabetes and the test for it – something that Bradford had recently introduced.

Some women present were doubtful and sceptical about the test. One in particular was quite angry about the way she and her parents had been treated in the past, and was adamant she would take no test because it would put her on a pathway that would stop her having the birth she wanted but have no actual effect on the outcome. Julie said nothing; she did not defend the policy, she simply listened to and acknowledged the concerns. These women were so impressed.

As she left, one of them said to me, "She listened. Until today, I have never met a midwife who could listen without interruption."

It restored her trust in the profession.

My trust in Julie's leadership and that of Consultant Midwife Alison Brown was so great that at a very difficult and precarious moment, I went to talk to them about information I had, trusting them to use it with the care and sensitivity it required. We were also able to have a very important conversation about the difficulties and challenges of implementing continuity of midwifery carer in the current structures. I took what I was told on board – we had shared values and aims – and it enabled me to understand better the challenges they faced and the concerns they had. This was extremely important for the coming months: I value the trust we shared on that day for that hard conversation.

It is not stylish leadership, it is not leadership with fanfare and pizazz, it tends to not get accolades, but it is leadership that builds trust and cooperation, that invites collaboration, and ultimately gets things done because of the diverse team working together with her. Too many NHS managers think it is all about them, and, as a result, they cause much suffering and resentment in women and indeed, their own staff. They also make mistakes because they don't have a team of people (including service users) telling them what is going on, rather than what they want to hear. The truth is that it is all about us: we can make this work TOGETHER. Julie and Alison understood that.

The Moral of This Tale:

- Cooperation across professional boundaries takes a style of leadership that values cooperation; it is about ending the them/us dynamic and making it all about 'us'.

- Good leadership in maternity – whether from the Head of Midwifery or the Chair of the MSLC or the leader of a campaign group – requires the ability and willingness to listen and see another point of view, especially when what is being said is difficult to listen to or something you would strongly disagree with. Remember, what you may find difficult to hear may give you the insight to avoid a mistake, a political faux pas or unnecessary conflict.

- Mutual trust and cooperation across professional boundaries can enable positive successes like the birth centre. It can head off conflict and difficulty, as you will learn in the next chapter, and it can enable communication in the midst of conflict and challenging situations that may mitigate or resolve the situation. Trust should be nurtured and treated like gold in maternity services.

- For NHS managers and campaign leaders, there is also a lesson to be learnt about not tarring everyone with the same brush. Stereotyping is so easy to do and prevents cooperation, by treating people as if they are your perception of the stereotype – this is the classic them/us paradigm.

Good leadership sees beyond stereotypes to work with real people open to partnership. This is the 'all about us'/'we can do this together' paradigm that maternity care should be all about.

Chapter 9

~⚬~

Working With Potential or Actual Conflict

THIS IS THE DIFFICULT ONE. If you want change to happen, if you hold organisations and leaders to account, if you are going to be any kind of activist, you will at some point find yourself in a conflict situation. It is said in activist circles that the first barrier you will face when you challenge an organisation or leader is indifference – you will be ignored, fobbed off, told lies, or mocked. If they start taking your challenge seriously, then you will enter a period of conflict. If they feel really threatened, it will stop being about the issue of contention over which they argue and they will focus their attack on you (cue the absolute incredulity and surprise of good midwives suspended after they raise concerns about practice or policy, or act outside guidelines to save a woman's life). It is usually after this particularly uncomfortable episode from the activist's point of view that the organisation will give in or come up with a compromise. In the stories you have heard in previous chapters and the ones that follow, you will see this pattern play out in various ways.

The Moral of This Tale:

- **If or when you find yourself in such a place of conflict, it can be hard, it can be messy, and it can be scary, but stay focused, stay rooted in your beliefs and values, be very alert to how you may be attacked, and have some countermeasures ready. Finally, be confident (whatever you feel), and don't blink first. You can do this!**

- **You don't have to do this alone. Seek out support of different kinds, from friendship, strategy meetings, paid therapy, to good legal advice.**

- **Conflict is not always negative: it can help sharpen your argument and hone your skills.**

- **Don't get deflected by high emotion – yours or theirs. See beyond the fireworks to what is the heart of the problem.**

Resolve It Privately if You Can: The Doula Problem

Whilst I was Chair of MSLC, doulas were being used more and more by mothers. Many of the doulas were friends or respected members of my network, and the parents who used them often came to the Choices group I ran or the breastfeeding groups I went to. Some mothers were so traumatised and upset by the unresolved experiences of their previous birth and the care they did or did not receive, that their solution was to employ doulas to be the trusted skilled companion at their birth where it was made clear to them there would be no midwife they knew and trusted attending. Some mothers would not allow the midwife/stranger into her birthing space unless necessary, and doulas were employed to protect their space and vocalise their decisions, and so were caught in the middle of the ensuing row about the role of doulas as advocates for their clients wishes.

The matter came to a head in that all too dangerous space at the end of the meeting: AOB. The Head of Midwifery, whom I respected, raised her concern about reports made by her midwives that doulas were overstepping their role. I could see where it might lead (doula bashing without knowing the whole story is very easy, as easy as midwife bashing, in fact), so I closed the discussion down before it had barely started: thanking the HOM for raising this important issue, asking if we could discuss the matter further after the meeting, and saying that we would report to the next meeting, which we did.

In my view, it would be no good having a "she said/he said" debate across the professional and competitive divide. There had to be a safe place of mutual trust and respect where concerns could be shared and mutually acceptable solutions found to the dilemmas these two sets of professionals faced in the birthing space.

I set up a private meeting in my home, in a quiet, calm, gently lit room where we would not be disturbed or overheard. In the event, it was the local doula network co-ordinator and a senior midwife who met with me in that room for the initial conversation. Both the women commensurate with their roles had prepared what they wanted to say. But then there was a space to talk around the issues and start finding solutions. Information was shared that meant they needed to go and find out more and have discussions with colleagues. It went so well that the meetings continued for some time without me needing to be there.

What had threatened to become a row and possibly a doula-bashing exercise – noticeably not a woman- bashing exercise, even though it was the women employing doulas to advocate for their choices – was averted by quiet private diplomacy. Indeed, better than that, an avenue of communication was opened, a safe space to discuss the difficult cases that inevitably occur in this arena. And it worked because I was respected by both parties, and I respected both parties. It worked because they agreed to meet privately on neutral ground and listen to one another, however difficult that may be. And I think it worked because of the people involved. In particular, the senior midwife who came had been an independent midwife herself and so was well aware of the challenges faced by advocating for decisions women make which go against accepted practice.

The Moral of the Tale:

- Try to resolve possible conflicts quietly and privately. Once it is in public, there is ample opportunity for insults, prejudice, personal vendettas and petty politics to come into play – some of which has nothing to do with the actual issue needing to be resolved.

- In most situations, there is a common ground where trust can be built and negotiations can be made – in this situation, the common ground was a common concern for the well-being and choices of the mother.

- All the stakeholders must come to the meeting wanting to find a solution and find a way of becoming allies across the boundaries. This is absolutely imperative to success.

- The private meeting should be in a neutral, private place where no one can listen in and where the meeting is undisturbed – safe for all parties therefore.

- Good tea or coffee and biscuits or cake are often helpful – actually essential! – especially in women's meetings. They act as a social facilitator – a shared pleasurable experience that is non-threatening to all parties.

- Sometimes it is helpful to have a skilled facilitator respected by the different parties, but this is not always necessary if the protagonists are motivated to find a resolution.

- It is really important that each stakeholder is given the opportunity to express their concern/position in a measured way, but also uninterrupted. Listening to and understanding the situation from the other person's point of view is the first step to finding a resolution in the interests of all sides. However, this also requires each party to express their position or concerns in a way that the other side will be able to hear. For instance, expressions of sadness and disappointment tend to work better than anger, measured language and nuance work better than bold statements of opinions, 'rules' and 'facts'. I had to do this recently and my inner mantra was "Speak with kindness because one day you could be in their shoes".

- Remember, people tend to do business with people – so pick your representatives with care.

Good Cop/Bad Cop

Good cop/bad cop is a game that Hospital Trusts have played on me and a game that I have played with them, as you have read. It is a team game where one half of the team say all the difficult things, are awkward, angry and provocative. The other half of the team are conciliatory and helpful, putting forward suggestions to resolve the issue which can in fact be the things they are willing to settle for. It can be quite fun to play (although in MSLC meetings, it was not fun to chair), and it is worth learning, even if it is only so you can spot when it is being played on you.

It can also work in a difficult meeting where you or your colleague are the focus of difficult, unacceptable stuff such as accusations of bad conduct, bullying, etc. Below is my good cop/bad cop story which was just such a scenario.

When the Shit Hits the Fan

As Chair of the MSLC, I had been trying to have a serious conversation with the commissioners about using continuity of midwifery carer throughout the maternal pathway to improve outcomes, women's satisfaction with the service and reduce infant mortality. I had significant medical evidence on my side and Bradford had one of the worst infant mortality rates in the country. However, I could not get a meeting with a decision-maker. My emails were not answered, my phone calls were not returned. I tried every ruse I could think of to find a way in, using friendly GPs, councillors, etc., etc., etc., but no one would talk to me or anyone in the MSLC about reducing infant mortality. Please note from the chapter's introduction that this is the first phase of opposition to a challenge.

Then One to One Midwives, an independent midwifery practice working wholly within the NHS, moved into the area, delivering exactly this kind of care to any woman referred to them. The health commissioning body were incensed and 'surprised' and cast about for people to blame – turning on me. After months and months of refusing a meeting about implementing continuity of carer, suddenly they wanted a meeting with me to discuss my poor conduct. Of course, they did not want to tell me the real reason – a tactic I was not going to put up with! I probed (via email) and eventually they admitted it was to do with my financial links with the midwifery practice because obviously if I was supporting a practice that delivered evidence-based care with the best outcomes for women and was what women wanted, I MUST have financial links with them! My response was to send 'one of my letters' which refuted the accusations and also issued my own accusation. Here is the gist of it:

How dare you assume that I do this for money! What kind of people are running our health service when they accuse someone paid almost nothing by the Trust, known to be fully committed to the delivery of the best maternity care and the best outcomes for women, of acting for money.

I copied all the MPs into the letter and anyone else I thought relevant. It was an indignant public refutation: I wanted to shame them, which I did, because the accusation was never mentioned again – it ceased to exist!

The Moral of the Tale:

Stay steady and stay rooted in your convictions and values, and think of the best way to ensure accusations such as this are openly (and publicly, if necessary) shamed and refuted. However uncomfortable it is, it has to be done. Friends who have tried to quietly and tactfully respond to such outrages have been taken down by their employer/opponent. You may be taken down anyway, but in my view, if I am going to go down, I am going to take them and their reputations down with me! Anyway, if you make the cost of pursuing spurious accusations very high they will, as in this case, back off.

But I still wanted that meeting! So a private meeting was agreed in a neutral place of my choosing but acceptable to the CCG as a meeting place they used too (see previous about finding a neutral safe space). I took someone into the meeting to be the 'good cop' (because I was clearly not going to be that!) and briefed her thoroughly on how the meeting probably would run and what we wanted from it.

The brief was:

- The CCG lead will want to shout at me (which they did) but they won't be able to do more than that because they don't employ me.

- We have lost the battle over the independent practice delivering the care we want for women, so we will let them run that. But we will push very hard with the medical evidence, the need to reduce infant mortality and morbidity, and what women want in regard to continuity of midwifery carer. We want commitments from them to deliver this themselves.

- But we have not got a guaranteed future for the MSLC, so we are going to make sure we get it, because in the long term this is the continuing opportunity we have to push for change. The key argument for the MSLC was: you need a stakeholder meeting with service users with knowledge of what is happening on the ground and in the community because if you don't, something like this [terrible political mess] could come and bite you on the bum again!

- The prize they get for playing our good cop/bad cop game is me stepping down from the position of Chair of the MSLC in the medium term.

I was obviously the bad cop so I sat meekly whilst being shouted at (and I was literally shouted at) and then we went to work, I pushed hard and let my colleague be conciliatory and helpful (which they lapped up). And at the end, I pointed out what a good Chair of the MSLC my colleague could be and that I was intending to stand down once this piece of work to sustain the future of the MSLC had been completed (big carrot left dangling). And the whole thing was wrapped up: we had turned a challenging confrontation into a win. We did not win everything we could have wanted but we got the MSLC and a verbal commitment to continuity. I generally think verbal commitments are not worth the paper they are not written on but it was something to push for in the continuing MSLC.

The Moral of the Tale:

- **I was shaking like a leaf going into the meeting. I was so scared! But focused, rooted in my convictions and values and having a strategy for the meeting, we played our game with gusto and won what we wanted with a few extra points on the side.**

- **Being shouted at because that is all someone can do to you, is not that big a deal when that is all they can really do to you and you have prepared for it as part of your strategy.**

- What I did not get from that meeting was a really good set of notes that I could wave in front of their faces for the following three years; my friend, the good cop and note-taker, did not furnish me with them afterwards. On the other hand, I was heading for burnout and was probably not able to follow them up in 18 months anyway. However, readers of this story, take note: make sure you record or take notes of all such meetings and have them sent round all the participants.

- Notes of a meeting in writing and agreed become the meeting record REGARDLESS OF WHAT ACTUALLY HAPPENED in the meeting. Anything not written down in the organisational world has not happened. If you can, take a scribe into any significant meeting for just this purpose.

- Sometimes an audio recording can be made. I don't think this meeting would have been one of those times. Where you are in fear of your job or reputation, then covert recording may be necessary. But either way, a good set of notes circulated trumps this strategically because people read and file minutes and they are easily circulated.

When the Shit Hits the Fan: Two Taps and a Plug Hole

This story is a good lesson in how, with some careful probing and negotiation, a large mountain can be reduced to a tiny mole hill.

I had a vision of making water birth a normal thing for women to do, and a birth bath to be a normal hospital provision. Indeed, I coined the word 'birth bath' because the birth pool was being turned into some mythical beast of high cost and technology when what it was in reality was a standard bath made big enough for a pregnant person to move around in and make themselves comfortable. What I should say in this context is that in order to do so in the UK, I had to break a monopoly.

Our prototype was made and we were beginning to market it when a solicitor's letter arrived. Our competitor was accusing us of copying their bath. And it was indeed a similar shape, because ovoid is a common shape, and indeed it did look similar in the way baths look similar – we had hoped we might be improving on the model.

There was an expensive exchange of solicitors' letters and then my dad suggested to me that rather than paying expensive solicitors, I should ring up and talk to our competitor to see if there was room for negotiation. I rang and listened long and hard to a very angry person, but then we began to slowly unpick the problem, to find the specific ways our bath might be perceived to 'copy' theirs.

At the end of perhaps the second or third long conversation, I put the phone down and turned to my husband saying,

"It's two taps and a plug hole! If we can move these, they will be satisfied."

So we removed the taps from the bath altogether and redesigned the plug hole completely (something that they also followed a while later but we did not accuse them of copying us!). And that was the end of it. Two taps and a plug hole. All that expense. All that anger and fear! Solved by moving two taps and a plughole.

Ever since then, when we are faced with a maelstrom of anger, bluster, accusation or complaint, whether it be in business, at home, as a Chair of a maternity committee or on the campaign trail, my husband and I will turn to each other and say, "*Two taps and a plughole!*" And in the vast majority of cases, with some careful listening and negotiation, we find that it boils down to this equivalent.

The Moral of the Tale:

- **Don't let the anger, emotion and threats of an opponent destabilise you. Probe and dig to find out what is really upsetting them and what a resolution might look like for them. It generally is far more mundane than the fireworks they set off suggest.**

- **And on the other side of the coin, in maternity services sometimes, in order to make some quite modest and basic changes, a massive, even spectacular, fuss has to be made! Once you have their attention, then the negotiation can begin.**

Conclusion

To summarise, if you are going to hold an organisation to account, challenge an injustice or make change happen, sooner or later you will find yourself in a conflict situation. All conflicts are ultimately resolved by some kind of negotiation or compromise somewhere. Finding a way to quietly and privately resolve a conflict is by far the best way, if possible, and I have provided some tips and ideas on how to do so. If you and your opponent can find a win/win situation where both sides feel they have been heard, have won something, and/or can save face – this is the ideal resolution.

However, if a person or organisation feels truly threatened, then do not be surprised if the attack becomes personal. In this situation, hold your nerve, stay focused and be clear-sighted about what is really happening behind the smoke and fireworks and bluster, then form a plan to resolve the situation using any tools and techniques you might find appropriate – I have offered you a few in the book.

Finally, beware of and be aware of personal attacks, and be ready to resist them robustly to protect you and your reputation, but be clever about it, because, as in judo, you can also use your opponent's outrage to further your cause.

Finally, we must understand that in a conflict situation, we can use all our skills and good heart to resolve the matter, but we should remember that we are not the only protagonists and so we cannot resolve the matter on our own – the other side must want to do so too. Particularly if the issue or row has moved into the public domain, other protagonists and political and financial interests may come

into play, preventing a resolution that benefits both sides –
it becomes a win or lose game.

In this kind of situation, we can play the game to the best
of our ability, but in the end we cannot always resolve or
win it. Do not take it personally, because the game is not
personal. Evaluate minutely what happened, learn from it,
move on.

Like the phoenix, you will rise.

To Conclude Part 2:
On Being an Activist

BEING AN ACTIVIST, and a birth activist, involves keeping a compassionate heart whilst playing political games of strategy and wit as intense as any game of chess or cards, but with much higher stakes. It can be fun, and it can be tough, it takes resilience, nerve and sometimes being downright bloody-minded. Nevertheless, the difference you make to the lives of dozens, hundreds, or even thousands of mothers and families, makes it worth the personal cost.

However, this is not everyone's cup of tea! Indeed, we need people who make tea and keep things going as an act of resistance whilst the row plays out! Nevertheless, no one can stay silent or inactive when they see poor care, poor practice and outcomes that betray a lack of care. In today's maternity system, sadly, we do not have to look very hard to find care that needs improvement, including the pay and conditions of midwives. To be silent is to be complicit and however uncomfortable it is, we are duty bound as professionals and human beings to act for the well-being of mothers and babies.

My advice would be to do what you can, find your allies so that the sum of the whole is greater than the individual, and fight clever to ensure that you get the best from the limited resources you have.

We need to be determined, clever, fun.

We need to band together to organise and unionise,

to write letters and demonstrate.

And we need to educate, educate, educate.

Talk to our daughters, sisters, mothers;

Talk to our sons, husbands, brothers;

And we need to fearlessly claim our heritage to birth and bring to birth,

To be the women, the mothers, the midwives we are.

We need to campaign as determinedly and creatively as we give birth,

Because our daughters are worth it

— and so are we.

Part 3

~

Activist Reborn

Chapter 10

❧

The Death of an Activist: Burnout

MY LIFE AS AN ACTIVIST crumbled slowly before suddenly collapsing with a couple of health crises. I call it the 'slow burn'. At first, I was too busy to be aware: I just felt tired all the time, and was breathless walking up mild inclines, the ducking and weaving, the bustle and excitement now wearied me. I did not want to do this anymore; I felt despondent and I began to think of succession. I began to put in structures and seek out people so that I could slowly begin to withdraw. I began to dream of living in a place where every encounter was not a conversation about birth. It was a long, slow process, perhaps taking three or four years.

And then, after a particularly challenging few months working, commuting between Wales and Bradford, and chairing the Parents' Association with a key role in the campaign to save our children's school, I felt TERRIBLE. It was 2016. A blood test showed my blood count was nearly half what it should be. My iron levels were brought back up to normal, but then dropped again when I tried to pick up my old pace of working. In the end, after a discussion with my family, I took a sabbatical of six months from both the business and activism. In those first six months, we lost the home we were renting and hoping to buy, and had to put most of our furniture in storage, with five of us moving into our tiny two-bedroom house.

The stress this caused had several unnerving physical effects but my medical herbalist checked me over and reassured me it was short-term stress. However, when I called the emergency doctor with rectal bleeding after a bowel movement a day or two later, he referred me to be checked out at a hospital.

When a few days later I called back to try and explain our stressful circumstances and ask if it could simply be a burst haemorrhoid (it was!), he shut me down and told me I had cancer. The shock of his words reverberated through the following weeks and through Christmas. It took four months to get the all clear – yes, it was simply a haemorrhoid caused by the stress of my circumstances. If only that GP had listened: he would have reduced so much of my suffering!

I was therefore not ready to go back to work after six months, so the sabbatical extended to twelve months, then two years, until I decided in February 2019 – or perhaps recognised – that I would not be able to work with that kind of stress anymore, even if I wanted to. Every time I picked up a campaign, after a few weeks it was too much and I had to drop it. A busy day in the office needed a day to recover. I resigned from being a birth activist and gave up the expectation that I could return to formal work patterns. My heavy, chaotic menstruation, which was probably the cause of the severe anaemia, stopped around the same time.

Then the world turned upside down as Covid-19 arrived, followed by lockdown in March 2020. My beloved father and trusted confidant died on a Covid ward in the first week of lockdown. Only eight of us attended the committal of his body and without all the comforts and support I had set up against this terrible day, I struggled to come to terms with this enormous loss.

As its contribution to the pandemic support, the Mindfulness Association[31] set up daily meditations. Dad had been a member of the Association and meditated twice a day; I saw daily practice as both support for myself and a connection to him. I had nothing else to do!

It was transformative. Slowly, very slowly, I healed. But I also learnt a way of living compassionately with myself as I am and being kind to myself and others. I practised new skills daily for living in difficult times. Five years later, I am finishing a book, thinking about what I do next and wondering if I might indeed find other ways to support women and midwives to change and disrupt the system that heals and hurts us.

Reflection

In his book *Recovery*, Dr Gavin Francis[32] talks about the use of the term 'breakdown'. He says that although it is not a medical term, there is a need for people to find a phrase, a descriptor for the personal cataclysm that has befallen them. Both burnout and breakdown as terms take us beyond the physical ailments that punctuate or perhaps usher in such a dark period, to reach into the mental and emotional breakdown, the hollowing out, the deep soul distress, the sense of having nothing left, no life left.

I have given a brief outline of my story above: it is not the purpose of this book to describe an anatomy of a burnout. Nevertheless, what we must do is acknowledge the fact and existence of burnout, how devastating it can be for the person and their family, and that it is a common affliction of activists on a particular campaign or generally. The causes and conditions of burnout and menopause are a political/ clinical book all of its own as well, so steering carefully, I want to reflect on what takes activists like me into burnout and what helps us to heal, recover and emerge to be active once more.

Menopause: Joining the Dots

As I listen to the stories of other women, it is becoming increasingly clear that menopause and its symptoms had a major role to play in what happened to me. If I had the knowledge and information 10 years ago that I now have, I would have made different choices, I may have avoided some of the worst effects that I suffered and it may have saved my business and activism. So many women like me have suffered extreme exhaustion, brain fog and memory issues, and with these can come depression and despair. It can last so long you come to believe that this is going to be the way it is forever and you might as well adjust your life accordingly, give up and resign from the things you once did so effectively.

It was only after I had passed through menopause that I heard the brilliant *Woman's Hour* series on menopause[33] and realised it could have been different. Listening a few years later to the brilliant *28ish Days Later* on Radio 4[34] gave me twinges of anger as women told my story back to me – of being at a peak in their career and giving it up in the middle of a menopause they did not know they were having. And finally, at a local WI talk on women's health, the dots were joined. I did not know what questions to ask, so I did not know what I did not know. And now I have to come to terms with the loss of a life I maybe need not have lost.

The red flags of poor care and decision-making are increasingly clear for me:

- I did not know, so I did not notice, in my busy life, the symptoms of perimenopause, in particular chaotic menstruation. I carried on coping without missing a beat until I was at the point of collapse.

- The GP practice handled the situation poorly, prescribing without discussion, explanation or even consent! The nurses booking the treatment appointments, confronted by a woman not willing to consent to anything without an informed discussion, first tried coercion. This was fatal for trust. Opportunities for helpful conversations were lost on both sides. After the 'cancer' debacle, I would not go near the practice for several years. Alternative medicine provided good treatment and support, but I look back and think a combined approach would have been more effective.

• Two questions that I asked repeatedly but were not picked up or dealt with and should have been. GPs would ask me if I had heavy menstrual bleeding – when I asked them to define what unhealthy heavy bleeding was, and how much it was, they could never say. This undermined my confidence in them because I had no benchmark to have an informed conversation. It was the medical herbalist that defined the term. I then immediately asked for help because I knew my bleeding was too heavy. The second question was mine: I felt very stressed and wondered if the heavy bleeding could be part of it (whatever it was, I was not sure). The standard response was, "What do you do for a living?" I would answer, "I run a business," and then they would change the subject as if I had never asked the question. I still don't know why they asked what I did for a living and why I received that response. I was terribly stressed and I felt I was going to break into pieces – but the conversation was closed down.

• Interestingly, a few years later on a mindfulness course, a man 10 years into recovery from a breakdown told me how he had been in hospital with a mental crisis when the doctors asked him what he did for a living. He told them he worked in construction and their response was to blank him and walk out of the room! He was as incredulous as I was; our experiences validated each other. My father, who had suffered two nervous breakdowns and years of depression, commented, "Ruth, medicine is very bad at dealing with mental health. They don't have the time or the energy to explore this with you." How true that was!

The Moral of This Tale:

- Before you reach the age of 45, make sure you understand fully the journey of menopause. Listen to *28ish Days Later*, to the *Woman's Hour* series on BBC Sounds, and other such podcasts. Learn from the stories of women who are living through it so you can devise your own path. It can be a path of suffering but it does not have to be; it can also be a journey of immense opportunity. And much of the suffering can be mitigated if you know where and how, and the health gatekeepers open the door.

- Those of us who have suffered or sailed through menopause need to share our stories, tips and thoughts so that the women who come after us are better prepared and can make the best choices for them.

- Don't give up. Find the practitioners, in both conventional and alternative medicine, who can support you in this transition. It is hard when you become as ill as I became, but they are out there.

- I have learnt only recently about how the hormones that guide your menstruation also control your ability to deal with stress: specifically that the decline of oxytocin and progesterone in menopause lowers women's resilience to feeling stress[35]. This explains clearly why I suddenly found myself unable to live with the same levels of stress I once had, and to live and work the way I once did. My 'buffer' has to be broader now. It would have been so much easier to have known this earlier so I could have made changes proactively before the crunch came...

- Like birth, there is no one-size-fits-all for women and menopause; medicine, society and women themselves need to acknowledge this truth and to allow each other to pick and choose their own path. It may well combine medical support with alternative and complementary medicine, counselling, diet and fitness, which is all good.

- Medicine needs to wake up to the responsibility of providing for the health needs of menopausal women and to make sure that women and health professionals join the dots so that appropriate care and interventions can be offered. This did not happen for me.

The Wintry Odyssey

Conventional medicine felt like it had little or nothing to offer me in my suffering so I lost trust in it altogether and began a journey, which now feels like an odyssey through a wild and wintry landscape. I started running and spent hours alone in wild places. My favourite place was in some woods by a river; I would just sit and watch it flow by for hours and it seemed to ground me, nourish me and, in some way, begin to knit me back together again. I could not read anymore – it was too much – so books, emails and all social media had to be abandoned. Social interaction and company were stressful and so were severely limited.

Except for my family. In the small world I now inhabited, my family became the front and centre of my life. During this time, I rediscovered my wonderful children: I treasured getting to know them again, I learnt how much I had missed them – and they had missed me: just by having my listening ear, my attention, my presence. I treasure the time we have spent together. I treasure the unconditional love and support they provided, their acceptance of me, even though I often felt I was useless and a burden on the family.

As my strength returned, but unable to deal with work and suffering from social stress, I decided to be the best homemaker I could be, caring for husband and family, doing the 'wifey' things – cooking, washing, gardening, being a listening ear – even cleaning (sometimes!). I had time to visit my parents and had some deep conversations which I now treasure. I have learnt that even in the most barren of life's winters, there are riches to be found, and this was indeed one of them.

For a couple of days a month, I started to go into the hills and stay in a cabin all alone: there was no Wi-Fi, no radio, no phone signal. I avoided what little human contact there could be. Being alone, being away from all social and media stimulation, this particular solitude has become a precious way of life: a turning within, a space without any obligations of time and relationship, a place to reflect and gain insight, to feel the feelings I have, to simply sit and watch the natural world and become part of it.

I had companions along the way. One was a precious yoga teacher and massage and reiki therapist, Juli Moran. She held my hand and was a guide through the dark and wintry landscape, teaching me skills to hear and heal myself. Becoming a Reiki Master is one of the precious gains of my wintry time.

The other guide was Tara Brach: to be more exact, her book, *Radical Acceptance*[36] – the only book I read in this period, and even then, very slowly. It became my handbook for healing, a map showing me paths through the wilderness, with stories of herself and others who had passed this way before me. Months stretched into years and I finally began to think I could find a quieter way of life but still a way of life that felt useful.

Covid-19 denied me my river and my cabin, and in my dad, the honest friendship of one person who knew my suffering, but I found the river and cabin within a daily practice of mindfulness meditation: a daily practice with others facing differing and similar challenges. This community has become a deeply treasured part of my life; our deep conversations nourish, guide and encourage me. Carrying your safe places inside you makes a massive difference to your resilience: I have grown stronger and more compassionate for myself and others through this practice and community. I have learnt a new level of kindness.

Like an addict, I can say now that I am in recovery, or like a cancer survivor, I am in remission. I work part-time on the business, I make fun forays into birth activism, but so far I have not ventured into any formal work commitment, partly because I am not sure I can take the pace and the stress anymore, and partly because having discovered family life, gardening and domestic joy, I am unwilling to sacrifice it all again. The vision still burns within but when I press on the accelerator, the power is no longer there like it was. My buffers must be broad. Wisdom and kindness must often suffice.

In her book *Wintering*[37], Katherine May interviews Dorte Lyager, a wild swimmer who talks about her way of surviving as a person with hypermania and depression. Lyager says:

> *"This has been a long journey for me, and swimming is just one of the changes I've made. I've cut out sugar, I make sure I get plenty of alone time, I go on long walks, and I've stopped saying yes to everybody. I've cut down my working hours. All of these things make a buffer, and I say I like to make my buffer broad. Sometimes problems come up that narrow that buffer, and then I have to make sure I build it up again. Keeping well is almost a full-time job. But I have a wonderful life."* (p210)

Lyager describes and affirms to me my own experience. I too have learned to live again as someone who was burnt out. My buffers are broad now and kept deliberately so.

Riding Three Horses With One Backside

Nevertheless, menopause cannot be blamed for everything. There are strong contributing societal factors which come from being a woman, a mother and an activist in the maternity system.

It has to be understood that along with my husband, we were bringing up five children, running a business that was beginning to internationalise, and I was an activist. So, on top of an already full life, I ran a monthly Choices group, I hosted a La Leche League group, I attended women's networking meetings to ensure maternity was on the city's strategic agendas, I was involved in countless groups and organisations on and off social media, I was Chair of the Committee that brought all the stakeholders in maternity together (MSLC/MNVP), and I was getting known as a speaker and Chair at conferences.

I was facing a huge amount of pressure so I had monthly physical and emotional therapy, weekly yoga or meditation classes, and we went away for a few days every couple of months to have a break. I set boundaries on my work in the office (although not in my head) and kept to them.

Nevertheless, I began to feel tired, weary even, and as I have described – it was not fun anymore. I was aware in the literature of pioneers and activists spending too long in post before handing on to the next generation, and I thought it might be time as I was so tired. I began planning succession so I could withdraw gently from some of the groups and responsibilities I had.

The La Leche League group left my home and flourished elsewhere. Choices groups were being set up around the area but I began looking for local leadership to ensure its continuity if I was not around. In particular, I looked for succession at the MSLC. I saw myself working more regionally and nationally, and decided I could not stretch myself any thinner between grassroots and strategic levels.

There is no career path for activists; indeed, a weakness of the maternity structures is that there is no pathway to use and retain expert representatives of service users. Once you have chaired an MSLC, where do you go? You have a mother with links into the birthing community, with years of in-depth knowledge of policy, evidence and maternity systems – do you simply let her go? And as a woman, where do you take all that knowledge and expertise? Particularly if that has led you into regional and national work. None of it is paid, or it is very poorly paid (small retainers do not pay bills!), so you have to rely on your partner's income or find paid work alongside your maternity work, whilst also raising your family. Is this right and fair? Furthermore, what a loss of experience and expertise to both mothers and the maternity services in general!

There comes a point, of course, when for many families this becomes unsustainable, and something has to give. I know women who have taken work way below their ability in order to continue their role as an expert maternity level representative at national level.

One woman is deeply respected – but unpaid, the only unpaid member of the committees – how wrong is that?! Another woman, a lawyer by training, now works as a low-paid care worker, because her decades of breastfeeding expertise, and editing national and international breastfeeding journals, provided no income, and she missed all the career milestones that enabled her to move easily back into another paying career.

> **Reflection Point: Expert representatives of mothers and families in maternity should not be the only unpaid professional in the room – and that is what we often are: having to read all the papers, understand all the structures and the concepts, but not being paid a bean for our time, knowledge and professionalism.**

Therefore, there are three structural injustices here:

1. There is a massive undervaluing of the knowledge and perspective of the women/service users in the system. In a professionalised system, the mother's voice is devalued because professional service-user representatives – with both expertise and knowledge of mothers' experience of maternity from the mother's perspective and the maternity system itself – are unpaid and have no pathway or progress. The assumption in the system is that we are laypeople with low levels of commitment who will move back into our careers and families after a couple of years. However, the system requires a whole other level of expertise for service-user involvement which takes years to accrue. This contradiction presents as an injustice because the levels of knowledge, professionalism and commitment, though required, go totally unacknowledged and unrewarded.

2. One of the outcomes of the mismatch of assumption and reality in terms of representation, is that the woman's perspective is often lost from the system as the level of attrition in expert mothers is high. This means there is a data gap of women's experience and perspective at key decision-making levels. Caroline Criado Perez, in her book *Invisible Women*[38], is very clear about the consequences of such data gaps in healthcare – they lead to woman-sized gaps in healthcare systems through which women fall.

3. Women like myself discover, after some years, that they have sacrificed their families and careers with massive financial and social consequences because they have continued to represent mother's voices in the system without pay, because there is no pay and no progression! This reinforces the structural inequalities that women already face in our society, in the workplace and maternity system.

This is hugely and structurally discriminatory, denying women a strong and professional voice at strategic levels. It is reflected in policies, practices and priorities that hurt mothers and their families, meaning that, once again, 'women's work' is undervalued and goes unpaid and unrecognised. In our culture where money denotes value and status, the message could not be clearer!

As I write, I can hear some of my former professional colleagues in maternity management point out the number of user surveys they have taken part in, such as the 'walking the patch', 'the fifteen steps', and so on. These are all well and good, and not to be dismissed; however, they are often conceived, organised, executed and interpreted through the lens of professionals working in the system, rather than those using the services. Therefore, they miss the perspective and priorities of mothers and parents and ask the wrong questions. **This** is the data gap and it is vast.

Women's and other users' perspectives are missing from key strategic and policy-making bodies, and it shows. We already know from research that mothers view their care differently to professionals. For instance, the concept of safe childbirth is understood differently by the professional with their medical lens, rather than the woman or pregnant person with their broader personal, social, economic and cultural lenses.[39] What mothers and parents need in the system is representation by people who have been service users and work with service users who can represent the service-user's perspective independent of the medical system. These people will have a strong knowledge of the physiology of birth and be able to navigate the maternity system. It takes effort and ability to do this, and we need to acknowledge and reward it appropriately.

As I saw the cracks in my life, I decided to reduce my workload and shift my maternity work to strategic policy levels and preferably paid places. As my health deteriorated, I started to withdraw from my activities, both paid and unpaid. In the end, I had to withdraw from both paid and voluntary work entirely – I could not ride three horses with one backside through menopause. I burnt out.

Chapter 11

❧

Born Again: Activism beyond Cynicism

I BEGIN THIS CHAPTER the day after the Ockenden report[40], the independent review investigating baby deaths over a 20-year period at Shrewsbury and Telford Hospital Trust. And my reaction is revealing to me of my current condition. Scrolling Facebook the day before, I note a post on the only birth activist group I now subscribe to, 'March with Midwives': it says that we all know that the publication of the report will be triggering and distressing to many people on the group, both mothers and midwives, and this is acknowledged and the group will be a safe space for people to express their grief and anger. With this early warning, I immediately decide to limit contact with the outside world for the next 48 hours or so. I do not go on social media, I won't read the papers or listen to the news. I am dealing with the grief of a family tragedy at the moment. I do not need this in addition.

But, of course, I cannot quite manage it! The following day, I risk listening to Radio 4's *World at One* whilst making lunch and am enraged by the "How could we know! How shocked we are!" apologetics and hand-wringing. When Prof Lesley Regan, then President of the Royal College of Obstetricians and Gynaecologists, is interviewed, I can barely listen and start shouting at the radio!

"I warned you five years ago!" I shout. "I wrote to you and told you there were serious issues when you were doing your confidential investigation and you never answered me!"

By teatime, my husband is suggesting, "If you are so upset about it, write to *World at One* and tell them." Can I find the letter I wrote, I wonder? (I lost many of my archives during my burnout.) In fact, it was relatively easy to find. The final sentences read:

> *If women are not being listened to, midwives not being listened to, tall poppies are bullied and disciplined – is the RCOG able to uncover these issues and ensure safe, evidence-based care is provided, to ensure healthy women stay healthy, and those with special needs are properly cared for?*
>
> *We are sure that, in due course, these serious flaws will come to attention. We are massively fearful of another Morecambe Bay in Shropshire and we once again write to you to ask that yourself and the RCM raise the alarm before things get worse.*

Five years ago, I along with others had raised serious concerns about the treatment of midwives who raised concerns with senior management. Five years before the Ockenden report was published, I raised the serious concern that the RCOG investigation was deliberately omitting to speak to the mothers who had organised themselves to protest at the closure of the midwifery units, whose stories revealed concerning details of poor care and practice.

For instance, what kind of care is being delivered when a mother describes the midwifery-led unit postnatal care as, "Putting me back together again so I could care for my family, emotionally and physically."

My fear was that if someone did not listen to and act on what these bullied midwives and ignored women said, there would be a 'Morecambe Bay'[41] level scandal at Shrewsbury and Telford. There is no triumph here in being right. Simply the raging impotent roar of the ignored. I don't get to challenge in public, the complacent apologetics of organisations that ignored the uncomfortable stories and concerns of women and midwives five years before. I weep and grieve for the harm done to so many, the injustice meted out to courageous midwives as yet unmitigated because they, and we, are not listened to. My head hurts with banging it against the brick wall of indifference: I go to bed with a heavy heart.

The following morning, I begin the emotional and mental repair; kind friends who know my background ask tentatively how I am, and listen respectfully to my rage. I sit in meditation and remind myself that I have a clear conscience; I did what I could then: struggling with my own mental health as I was, I wrote to everyone and warned them. I supported a midwife suspended on trumped-up charges for speaking out about her concerns. I could do no more. Even now, I have found the letter I sent to the

Chief Executive of RCOG and forwarded it to *World at One* asking them to challenge the organisation further. I no longer have the emotional resilience to do more than that, but I have done what I tell others to do:

"Do what you can. You don't need to do more."

This is a really important lesson – to do what you can and accept that. Remember, where true guilt resides is not with you.

I remind myself that this suffering is from compassion for others and that compassion must also care for me. So finally, I can hug myself and weep, as I weep now writing this.

The price of caring, the price of my activism, is invisible impotent grief because I can see the harm being done, but can do nothing to prevent it. It is like those horrible dreams I have sometimes where I scream for help, but no sound comes out. Nobody hears me.

We all know this is not a unique experience. Men and women over decades and centuries have shared my impotent rage. Jonathan Freedland in his book *The Escape Artist*[42] tells the story of the man who memorised every detail of the killing machine of Auschwitz, then escaped to warn the world. Freedland details the fury he carried the rest of his life, because no one took him seriously and so many millions more suffered and died.

So this chapter must begin to face the difficult reality of powerlessness and impotence, of being a woman and a birth activist in a patriarchal, factory-based system, which you are unable to completely change (even if you make changes), and finding a way to survive it. There are two different paths to go down.

The Path of Analysis to Action

Firstly, the path of socio-eco historical analysis that unearths the causes and conditions that make change in maternity services so difficult. Interestingly, it was from the strong social justice tradition of my Christian faith that I learnt and practised this path, following a biblical and Christian tradition of compassion for all God's children and a conviction that everyone deserves justice and kindness. My theology and church history degree taught me to question everything, both fact and opinion, including every aspect of my own faith and convictions:

What is the evidence? What is the motivation or interest of the speaker? Why is this being said in this time and place?

In the humanities, there is no such thing as impartiality – it is a myth: there can only be awareness of your own and others' bias and 'baggage' (that is your family, your education, your life experience, etc.).

This learning was finely honed by the study of liberation and contextual theologies. The methodology developed was rooted both in experience and action alongside research and analysis.[43] It runs like so: a simple experience of injustice might be selected or might be a trigger for analysis and action, such as the moment a qualified midwife defers to a doctor to say whether I am fully dilated or not during my first birth. Then comes the analysis using all the tools of historic, economic and social critique and analysis to look at where the power lies, in whose interest is the situation played out and why, what are the structures that underlie this event, and provide the cultural, political and economic context. In the case of this small cameo, it could be the lack of the autonomy of the midwife rooted in the socio-economic position of women historically, the history of obstetrics as a male-only profession set up to dominate and control both women's bodies and the female professionals that cared for them. We can see this currently played out in the differential pay between obstetricians and midwives, the status and control consultant obstetricians and clinicians hold within the maternity and hospital system, which makes our midwife fearful of her own professional expertise. And we see the impact on me as a woman, at the bottom of the power hierarchy, having to 'wait for a doctor' before being allowed to birth my baby – infantilised and without autonomy.

In Christian and other faith liberation methodologies, we would then seek out biblical or equivalent 'antecedents':

Where have women or other disadvantaged groups faced injustice? What did they do about it? What was the outcome?

So for my story, I might recall, for instance, the two midwives to the people of Israel enslaved in Egypt who were commanded to drown all the male babies by their Egyptian overlords (Exodus 1:15-20).[44] They refused to do so, and when challenged, replied that the women of Israel were strong, healthy women who birthed quickly and so the babies were born before arrival (BBA) of the midwife! It could be seen as a courageous act of subversion.

I might reflect on the Syro-Phoencian woman in the Gospels who asked Jesus to heal her son. Jesus dismissed her request with what we might now refer to as a racist trope, her witty comeback called his bluff and changed his mind (Mark 7: 24-29).[45] This may have been a light-hearted exchange or been a sharper battle of wit, but nevertheless as a non-Jewish woman she was talking back at a higher-status Jewish male: a courageous and witty word of challenge to power.

The fourth stage in this methodology is action: *What can we do about it? What shall we do about it?*

In the liberation practice, there is always action to follow analysis – it is never ever simply an academic book-based exercise! So what did I do? Well, this book tells the story! However, as each action is taken, the methodology loops round again. For instance, I tell the story at a conference providing the analysis above and calling for action, my speech is then printed in the AIMS journal, so I have publicly raised the issue and taught the method of analysis and action.

What happens next? Using the same tools as above and the same process, the next action is planned and executed. And so there is constant reflection, evaluation and action taking place, rooted in a set of values and a community who both support and restrain.

On a personal level, this enables us to see clearly the macro gender and socio-economic structures at play which define our experience and our sphere of influence and action. It enables us, for instance, to understand that it is not our fault; that our experience and lack of power is anchored in structural gender-based discrimination which will take generations to overcome. This puts our actions – both failures and successes – in their proper context and makes it clear that we are responsible only for what we can do – not for what we can't, nor for what others do or don't do.

The Moral of This Tale:

- Taking time to analyse the issue enables us to see clearly its causes and conditions.

- Analysis and action-reflection methodologies enable us to plan our strategies effectively.

- If you have a belief or value system, it can strengthen and inform this process.

- However, we have a limited sphere of action and influence.

- We are only responsible for what we can do for change.

- We are NOT responsible for what others do or don't do.

The Spiritual/Mystical Path of Action

Alongside the first path is a second path, which can be both mystical and spiritual. It is where we come to terms with the suffering of both others and ourselves, and learn compassion and acceptance which enables us to carry on taking action with the clear-sighted understanding that what we do may feel futile and may actually do very little to change things for the better. We do it because it may help and because it is the right and compassionate thing to do.

Maiden, Mother, Crone

In the old traditions, there are three stages in a woman's life: maiden, mother, crone. The **maiden** is the young and beautiful woman with life before her, when all is possible and dreams are dreamt and plans are made. The **mother** is the one who has given birth to these possibilities, whether they be children, a career, the care of others, or all three. She slogs away to make her dreams come true, heart and soul, wanting to see her offspring reach maturity and deriving great joy as they do, and much grief where they do not – for she loves them all as herself. The **crone** is the elder, the one who has passed the menarche, whose dreams and possibilities have grown up and moved on, or have sickened, died and been mourned for. These women have seen both success and failure, the joy of productivity and the searing grief of loss; they have possessed beauty and agility and watched it change and fade. They now accept it all as part of life; and from that acceptance, there comes wisdom and a kind of earthed serenity.

And so I see in my life, and those of other women, three phases of activism. As young activists (maidens), we see wrong and harm, and with energy, passion, creativity and belief, we set about changing the world – because we believe it can be changed, and indeed it can.

As we become the mother, we take on the hard work of making our ideals work in reality, giving our time and talent to committees, taking on roles, organising, speaking truth to power, holding to account, fundraising, and, importantly, making change happen. We build our new world with pride for our daughters to enjoy, pouring our heart and soul into the work until we have nothing left to give. It is at this point that the tragedy of our situation becomes apparent as we watch what we worked so hard for being undermined, attacked, dismantled, destroyed. It is heart-breaking, and literally soul-destroying.

When we accept we have nothing left to give, when we finally accept reality as it is, when we know who we really are – both our power and our impotence – when we can continue to do what we can with what we have, in the full knowledge that tomorrow it may also be lost, when we can encourage and nurture and seek to protect the young activists rather than envy or undermine them, then we are the crone – for we have found a place of wisdom and a kind of earthed serenity.

Here is an account of my crone-dom:

My Grieving Soul

And so I see the Maiden
Held by her Mother
Crying in the sunshine.

I watch the Mother
Held tightly in the arms of her Love
As she sobs

And I the Crone, sit,
feet dangling in the stream
watching the water flow from me
making its way to the ocean.

I sigh.
Time to return home
To finish making that shawl
To cover my shoulders.
To wrap around
my grieving self.

It is important to understand that no one gets to skip these phases of life and of activism – unless you give up or die. Just as the sun rises and the seasons change, we change and move on as we live life. It is also important to understand that there is nothing deficient about being the person in each of these phases; one is not better than the other; indeed, I think sometimes we may be more than one at a time. All are necessary in the fight against injustice, all of us have a role in making change happen and repairing the harm done by ignorance and systemic injustice, and all of us support and care for one another so the sum of us is greater than the individual.

Beyond Cynicism

As a young activist and community organiser at the Urban Theology Union (UTU), John Vincent, founder of the UTU, teacher and mentor, would state often and repeatedly that failure was integral to activism. Most of the time you fail, he would say, and most of your successes will be dismantled within a generation, for someone else to have to re-imagine and rebuild. Don't become a social entrepreneur or a community activist if you are not prepared to fail because failure is the norm. This was extremely useful advice and although I took it with a big pinch of salt at the time, it ensured I did not take inevitable failure personally. Except that, in the end, I did, not because of the failure to change things per se, but as with the launch of the Ockenden report, the deep grief of seeing harm being done but being unable to stop it – with all the will in the world. It is now called **Moral Injury**.[46]

Ian Duffield, a colleague and tutor alongside Vincent for many years, reminded me of this as I discussed with him the unfolding tragedy of living long enough to see a new generation of mothers having to fight exactly the same battles as I did! He said there are three ways people meet this kind of reality:

1. You give up and forget it.

When I burnt out, this is what I did. This is what many mothers and midwives do. We cannot do it anymore, so for our own well-being, we walk away. There is another kind of giving up too: those who have resisted the system give up by giving into the system and conforming to it, colluding with it, advocating for it, because it is simply easier and more sustainable to do so.

2. You are driven into cynicism.

The cynic is the one that says, "It is not worth doing anything because nothing really changes," "They are all the same," "It won't make any difference whatever I say or do." It is heard in the mouths of midwives who dismiss mothers wanting a physiological birth as 'white witches and social workers', or 'the usual hippy crowd'; and the people who take satisfaction or watch with glee as women and people try and fail to wrest control of their birth from the system.

3. You go beyond cynicism.

When we go beyond cynicism, we see what the cynic sees but choose to respond differently. We carry on acting with compassion and acting to disrupt and change systems that harm. We do this knowing that our success may be limited, that it may be dismantled, that we might face opposition, that we may fail. But we do it anyway because for us, it is the right and compassionate thing to do and maybe this time we will ultimately succeed. Beyond cynicism, there is always hope because as we act and speak out, we make space for others to do the same. When we show compassion and kindness, we are rewarded with human connection, solidarity and relationships to treasure, as well as beautiful births and happy babies. Going beyond cynicism is an act of radical love in the face of a system that can harden us, an assertion of our humanity in a system that can all too easily strip us of our humanity.

When I look back over the work I have done over many years with clear-eyed honesty, I can see what we achieved being dismantled. And I can count the cost of the many hours, the money spent, the difficulties overcome to make that change happen. As I write, the Bradford Birth Centre is robbed of its dedicated staff, regularly closed so staff can work on the Obstetric Unit. This demonstrates a senior maternity management who do not see the unit as essential to ensure (as per the evidence) that healthy women have physiological births and to keep healthy women from blocking obstetric beds in the obstetric unit. Friends in Bradford have described the birth centre as "closed more than it is open" – maybe it is time to do an FOI request to find out. But what this does do, is deny women the birth place choices recommended in Baroness Julia Cumberlege's

Better Births Report[47]. Speaking of Better Births, the national commitment to deliver continuity of midwifery carer to women has been rescinded, denying women and babies the evidence-based health benefits of a 'midwife I know and trust'. Independent midwives were not saved despite our best efforts, and lost their insurance[48] and with it, their right to attend any births (except their own). Meanwhile, the Parliamentary Report on Birth Trauma[49] has come out and the latest figures on maternal mortality show mortality rising, with black women and poor women suffering the most[50] – issues Better Births set out to tackle. The list goes on and on, and is so depressing.

Can I be cynical? **Yes, I can.** Am I angry? **Yes, I am.** Will I stop working for change? **No, I won't.** Because there is a new generation of mothers and midwives, with energy, enthusiasm, who are techno-literate and media savvy, picking up the baton. I follow 'March with Midwives'[51], 'Pregnant Then Screwed'[52], and 'Birthrights'[53] and more with a mixture of gratitude and respect. Whilst there are women and midwives willing to fight for the well-being of mothers and the autonomy of midwives, there is no reason to give up. Even if there is every reason to be realistic about achievements and cynical about political and managerial promises. After four years, independent midwives got indemnity insurance: although it is expensive, they are now attending births – wonderful news for mothers and their families! I am told by one campaigner that the commitment to continuity of midwifery carer is not yet lost beyond reinstatement, so watch this space. Going beyond cynicism means being clear-eyed about the odds but resisting anyway, out of compassion, because it is the right thing to do, and because we refuse to let hope die.

I recognise, since my breakdown, that I cannot go back to the life I once led, and for a while I did give up for my health and well-being. But now I have walked back into the arena, aware of the reality of my limitations and the overwhelming odds we all face, but I do it out of love and compassion for other mothers – my daughters and nieces, friends' daughters and nieces, my siblings worldwide. I do what I can.

The Guerrilla Activist?

What I can do, currently, is pick up an issue, such as mothers being denied the support of their partner during the pandemic when they are told their baby had died, or the sky-rocketing rates of induction at a single hospital, or a mother being told she cannot use the pool because there is a hole in it when the only hole is a plughole. I run with it using all my skills and experience, making as big a deal of it as I can and then after several weeks or months, I move on. I appear, sometimes unrecognised, until the proverbial hits the fan.

There was a small moment of glee when a Head of Midwifery sent a message after I made an anonymised complaint about 'the hole in the bath'. (A niece was told that she could not use the pool because there was a hole in the bath!) The message I received was that the matter had been reported to the manufacturer for them to rectify. To the parents of the other 5,999 births in that hospital, this would have closed the matter down, but I was the manufacturer and no one had reported a hole in a bath to me! It is a matter of fact that although the glaze can be cracked if something heavy like a spanner is dropped into our birthing bath, the on-site maintenance staff can repair it. It takes a sturdy drill to make a hole in one of our baths, which is what it takes to make the plughole. Anyway, I blew my cover and had the satisfaction of an uncomfortable Head of Midwifery swiftly trying to shift ground, having been caught out.

I had a conversation about 18 months ago with my independent midwife. It is a tribute to the true profession of midwifery that mothers like me decades later refer to 'my' midwife with the same respect as 'my mother' (sometimes more so). I told her how I had come to accept that I could no longer carry on sustained campaigns over months and years. All I could do, I said, was pop up for an intense burst of activity on a specific issue before dropping below the radar again. She observed that this was a powerful strategy.

"They don't know where you are. Ostensibly you have gone, but then all of a sudden, out of nowhere, you pop up and cause a fuss, then disappear again. No one knows where you are and where or when you might pop up next. How very unsettling for them!" she smiled.

Truly, I have become a guerrilla activist. Guerrillas are fighters who do not have state-sponsored personnel, weaponry and machinery. They have to use their knowledge of the land and people to appear and disappear at will, to attack and withdraw, attack and withdraw. I use my knowledge, skills and bloody-mindedness to kick up a fuss here or there but then as the wheel turns, I disappear again back into my quiet life. Disappear, but not quite gone; at any moment, I might pop up again and cause a stink for a few weeks before disappearing into the undergrowth once more.

Every guerrilla activist (and those who are not) must understand both the power and the limitation of this form of activism. It brings energy and flair to the long-rumbling discontent; it can shift the debate sometimes, but it is seldom long term and fully strategic: that is the role of others. High-energy action can seldom be sustained for a long time, especially when acting alone or in a very small group – but it can affect results where formal routes are blocked. The Suffragettes, XR, Insulate Britain, Just Stop Oil and so on, all take action in this tradition. In the Christian tradition, there is the concept of the Community of Saints; in Buddhism, there is the Sanga: an understanding that we are all connected, that our actions are part of a greater whole of which we are but a part, that working together connected and supportive of each other, we can effect change. Our different ages, roles, status, actions complement each other if we stay connected and compassionate.

What I am learning as I go beyond cynicism, is what every guerrilla activist needs to know: you are never on your own, there are always supporters – possibly under the radar because of their situation, but your loud voice gives cover for others to shout, and your small acts of resistance make space for others to push the door wider.

The Granny in the Kitchen

When my children were very small (so over a period of 10 years!), I took them to a well-run toddler group called See & Know which I ended up leading for a while. It was highly structured with an introductory free play time, followed by small groups with structured teaching and singing time, third came an activity, and finally, tea and juice and biscuits/ fruit with free play. It all took place over the course of an hour. The group was ostensibly led and run by mums who welcomed parents, and organised and led both the groups and the activity.

However, in the kitchen were 'the grannies'. The grannies set up and made and served the tea and fruit (as biscuits became outdated). They helped set up the hall beforehand and helped clear up after, and they turned up to the committee meetings that organised the programme. Once the tea was served, most of the grannies would wander into the hall and chat with the mums, listening sympathetically to tales of joy and woe, holding a baby whilst a mum popped to the loo, grabbing a runaway toddler of a nursing mum, quietly wiping away shed tears. Without ever giving advice, the grannies would share their experience, and so I along with other parents learnt that mums in another generation had suffered challenge and difficulty but had made it through to the other side. After chatting with one of the grannies, I always felt better, that I was an okay mum and I would be able to carry on being a good mum until I was out the other side. The grannies were older women in the church, mostly retired, whose children had grown up, and they often had grandchildren.

These women have become a role model for me of the other side of activism. The facilitators, the supporters, and the nurturers of whatever age or status. The people who turn up to meetings just to support, turn up to stalls and events, who set up the chairs and the kitchen, who bring cake, and wash-up and help clear up. The people who ring you up or check-in with you to make sure you are okay, and will provide a confidential listening ear and shoulder to cry on.

To be an activist and do all I did, I needed support: my husband making the tea every night and often putting the kids to bed, a staff member to cover the phones and do the admin so I could do my thing, the people who hosted meetings, made tea and brought cake.

Being on the front line can be brutal, so strategically as activists we need to ensure we support one another. It is not about actually being a granny, it is about acknowledging the importance of the role of supporter, nurturer and facilitator behind the scenes. Maybe we need to recognise the 'step forward, step back' nature of activism. Most of us cannot be on the front line forever so we step back and someone takes our place whilst we take on the role of supporter and nurturer. Certainly in these latter days, that is how I have come to see myself – providing support, encouragement, strategic insight and advice where wanted, to my children and anyone else, to be a person who understands and cares – so others can go out there and make change happen when I cannot.

There is a role in activism for the *granny in the kitchen* who makes sure the chairs are set up, provide tea and cake and a listening ear, and who clears up afterwards. It is essential to our well-being and survival, particularly in long drawn-out and sometimes brutal campaigns. I hope and aspire to be a *granny in the kitchen* in the coming years.

Lessons in Self-Healing and Survival

There is so much rubbish talked about resilience – often by employers inappropriately demanding more from their staff; but there is no doubt that mental and emotional well-being enables you to do more for longer as an activist. Resilience is not a magic pill that makes you immune for what is thrown at you, but it can help.

What I also know is that simply telling someone to be robust, to be compassionate, to not take it personally, is not enough – it often ends in suppression and projection, covering up your feelings, acting and masking, rather than being the precious human you are. What we need is to be told **how** to have robustness and compassion, to not take things personally, whilst not becoming hardened cynics or burnt-out wrecks: "tender and tough," as Maya Angelou says in her book, *Wouldn't Take Nothing for My Journey Now*[54].

In the last five years, I have read Tara Brach, Pema Chödrön, and more. During the pandemic, I became a member of the twice daily sits of the Mindfulness Association. I have been struck by the Tibetan Buddhist emphasis on compassion. Whatever you do, make compassion the centre of it, is the founding ethos of the organisation. I have also been struck by the Buddhist attitude to developing compassion and mental resilience. Their attitude is if you want to play the piano, you practise; if you want to be an athlete, you train; and if you want to be compassionate and mentally resilient, then you train and practise too. And so there are devised practices and training programmes to help us understand how our minds work[55] and to develop healthy and compassionate hearts and minds. It takes effort and practise to be systematically compassionate for everyone, including being kind to yourself, but the payoff is a game-changer. And for me, now post-burnout, it makes the difference between whether I can take action or whether I cannot.

Go find out about it and see if it works for you. Or find something else. But remember, it is not fairy dust; it may make you more resilient for longer, but practise may also tell you that walking away is the most compassionate thing to do for you and for others. Below I share practices I have learnt which nurture and heal and enable me to get involved again.

Drinking Tea with Mara

In the dark days of my burnout when I would get up, get dressed and eat breakfast, then go back to bed exhausted from the effort, I picked up Tara Brach's seminal book *Radical Acceptance*[56] which became my handbook for self-healing. From it, I learnt about 'Drinking Tea with Mara'. Mara in Buddhism is the being of hatred and war, fear, greed and so on, a near-equivalent to the Christian Satan. After the Buddha's enlightenment, when he had withstood a night of torment by Mara and come through to the morning steadfast and thus fully enlightened, it is said that Mara would still on occasion return to visit him.

When Mara appeared, his servant would say, "Shall I chase him away? Call guards?"

The Buddha would reply, "No. Show him into my tent."

And the Buddha would sit with Mara, offer him tea, and drink tea and talk with him. After a while, Mara would go away.

Drinking Tea with Mara. It caught my imagination: why not drink tea with those spectres that tormented me? So I decided to have tea with Mara. On a day when I was alone in the house, I made a big pot of tea, and took some milk and the kettle to my bedroom. And I Drank Tea with Mara. In my mind, I called to the table the feelings that haunted me – Grief, Anger, Fear, even Death on at least one occasion. Also, 'I Ought To.' I invited friends too: Jesus Christ, Dr Usui (founder of Reiki), Divine and Reiki Light, my dad.

I would turn to Fear and say, "You are in a safe space here, I am listening with open heart. Say what you need to say to me and I will listen."

And Fear would speak. There were tears and often I ended up having compassion for Fear, and Grief and Anger (or that part of me that are these things), because these feelings were so appropriate to the situation. Sometimes the friends would offer words of comfort but mainly they were a silent, supportive, protective presence. Over several months, I had several tea sessions but as I healed, I did not need the mammoth tea-drinking sessions anymore. But it remains one of my 'go-to' practices for rotten times. And I offer it to you as a possibility of listening to your own hurting self, and making peace with yourself. We are not broken and need fixing; we often simply need to listen to the hurting, angry parts of ourselves and totally accept them – and us – as we are.

The RAIN Practice

Tara Brach's RAIN practice is a handier, pocket-sized version of Drinking Tea ... which can be done on a walk, in the garden, or a half-hour timeout of a stressful or conflict situation. See *True Refuge: Finding Peace And Freedom In Your Own Awakened Heart.*[57]

First is **R** – Recognising the feelings inside you, maybe naming it/them with compassion and no judgement.

A is to allow their presence (like the return of Mara). This is the inviting them into your tent for tea.

I is Intimate Attention, when you listen to what your feelings are saying. If you have the chattering brain like mine, where the story becomes a loop or a tornado of words, it is important to drop below the words and story loop to the emotions underneath: *What am I feeling right now? What else am I feeling right now? Where do I feel it in my body?* Finding the anchors of our suffering beyond the words enables us to find the deep, hurting self, hidden by our stories: the self that needs comfort.

Finally, **N** for nurture. We give that hurting self some comfort: hand on heart, hugging ourselves, loving our hurting self, holding our hurting self with kindness without guilt or judgement, loving ourselves.

N is also sometimes termed non-identification – when we stop identifying with the problem. It is so easy to become what hurts us: *I AM angry, I AM sad, I AM overwhelmed.* If we can change those words to *I am FEELING angry, I am FEELING sad, I am FEELING overwhelmed*, this starts to put some distance between us and those feelings. It is like adjusting the lens from a single focus to a wide angle – this one thing is seen in the context of our whole life, the beautiful world we live in, the universe. It might be painful and overwhelming for us now, but it is also only one small segment of life and our identity. We can feel it and we can also let it go. It is a moment, however fleeting, when you see or observe yourself being angry, upset, etc. – at that moment, you are not the feeling, problem or the mistake. Whatever it is, it is not you, the real you, but happening to you, passing through you. It gives you some sense of distance, some sense of perspective, some sense that you are bigger than this thing. Remember, feelings happen to you – they do not define you.

Sometimes with this practice comes insight, but in any case, and indeed what is most important, is that we are showing the kindness to ourselves that we need – the kindness we would offer to a friend.

Here is how I wrote up a RAIN practice for the Ockenden report:

R

As I recalled what happened to me and to others
I felt ANGER.
No – not anger – but
FIERY INDIGNATION

A

"Drop the story," I said to myself, "and feel the fury."
Then I asked myself, "Is there anything wrong with this
feeling?"

"No," came the answer.
"Because this is an appropriate feeling for what happened and happens."
The insipient feeling of Guilt that had slipped into my soul, slipped out as I said this.

I

Then a huge blanket of fatigue settled upon me, throat constricted, heart heavy.
This was the powerlessness, the impotence, the inability to prevent harm and enact effective change. This was the feeling of it.
And I felt Compassion and Love for the Fiery Indignation, and also for me, and for everyone.

N

So there it was:
Fiery Indignation
Burning with a big flame
in the crucible.
And surrounding it
A beautiful circle of love and compassion
lit by the glow of the fire.

And I sat, holding the precious image,
and the sense of
Fiery Indignation held in the Cup of Compassion.

Love Is the Way: Loving Kindness Practice

Bishop Michael Curry quoted Martin Luther King at the wedding of Harry and Meghan, the Duke and Duchess of Sussex.[58]

"Love is the Way. When love is the way, then no child will go to bed hungry … when love is the way, we will let justice roll down like a mighty stream … when love is the way, poverty will become history … when love is the way, we will lay down our swords and our shields …"

This was no sentimental love; this was 'tough and tender' love, born from the suffering and activism of black African Americans. Activism out of a heart of compassion.

Thich Nhat Hanh was a Buddhist monk and peace and justice activist in Vietnam during the Vietnam war until he was exiled to France. In *The Art of Living*[59], he tells a story of hearing news of a Vietnamese boat being overrun by pirates, where a 13-year old girl was raped, murdered and her body thrown overboard. He was filled with impotent anger. And so he turned to his Buddhist practice, meditating all night. At the end of the night, he was filled with love and compassion, for the suffering of the murdered girl, the suffering and grief of her family. And because of his sustained compassionate practice, he felt compassion for the suffering of the pirate who committed the crime, to the point when he said, "If I had been born into that life and upbringing, I too might be a pirate."

Philip Yancey, in his seminal book *What's So Amazing About Grace*[60], tells a similar story in a Christian context when a young man's best friend is murdered in cold blood during the US civil rights campaign. In a heart-rending account, the young man not only found it in himself to forgive the perpetrators, but bought a farm and stayed in the area, becoming a "Minister to the rednecks" who had killed his black friend.

This is advanced practice both for Christians and Buddhists. It is about forgiving the unforgivable – not for their sake, but for ours. When unspeakably cruel wrong is done (e.g. the trauma report), we carry a huge burden of justified anger, grief, resentment and bitterness, However, the problem is it hurts us more than it hurts them, so we have to find a way of dealing with it. Advanced practitioners might quote Martin Luther King as above saying, "Love is the Way".

It starts with love for ourselves and compassion for the suffering we experience because of what happened. It also begins with an acceptance of the wrong that has been done, and an acceptance of ALL the feelings we have – and for a long time, this is all we can do. However, as we feel safe, held in that love and self-compassion (see the RAIN practice), we are able to reach out and touch the pain of others – sometimes only for a few minutes – but in so doing, we start making the kind of connections that with time and practice bring healing.

It takes practise to love like that. And it is likely that Thich Nhat Hanh, in his night-long vigil, used versions of two practices I want to share here, practices I use because they work: the Loving Kindness Practice and Tonglen.

The first enables my heart to open out in love for everyone because we are all human and it is difficult being human sometimes. The second practice enables me to be open to the suffering of others, stay soft and kind, whilst not becoming overwhelmed, embittered and hardened by it. They are practices because that is what we are doing – practicing so we can show love and compassion both to ourselves and to the suffering in the world we encounter. They never stop being practices because we never stop practicing!

So we begin.

The Loving Kindness Practice

Hand on heart, I would invite you to say these phrases quietly to yourself:

May I be well, may I be happy,

May I be free from suffering and live life with ease,

May I flourish and grow,

May I have joy without needing a cause,

May I be safe.

May I be filled with loving kindness.

Compassion begins with ourselves, so practicing compassion begins with ourselves. Saying the words may generate love within you or you may feel numb, or even irritated. That is okay. Note your feelings, but continue to say to yourself, *May I be well, may I be happy...*" etc.

It does not matter if it feels mechanical and wooden; words have their own power, so just roll with the practice.

Then we start wishing these good wishes for others. If we are on the go, we might do it for the people in the room or on the bus, or for the people we are about to meet, whoever they are. And I have found that simply wishing good things for others as well as myself, makes me feel calmer and happier. The classic practice, however, moves through seven levels of increasing difficulty and/or broadness, starting with someone or something which we find easy to love – and that is often not ourselves:

1. We wish good things for someone we love whose relationship is not complicated (as some close relatives or friends can be). It could be a pet or a child – someone for whom it is easy, really easy, to wish good things for. It is the feeling or the sense of loving kindness we want to recognise here, so that what we feel for someone or something we find easy to love can then be replicated for ourselves and for others.

2. We wish good things for ourselves, affirming our own worth (however we feel about that at the time). It can be difficult for some of us sometimes to feel love and acceptance for ourselves, so say the words of loving kindness and accept the feelings as simply being what they are.

3. We wish good things for someone we are close to, maybe a more complex or mature relationship.

4. We wish good things for a neutral person, like the bus driver, or shop worker, or someone we see around but don't know. Here we are broadening the scope of our compassion and empathy beyond our own small universe.

5. We wish good things for a person whom we find difficult. And this can be very difficult to do so don't pick your most difficult person on your first few goes – work up to it. Also work with compassion for yourself. Don't do too much all at once; recognise anger, irritation and so on in yourself and accept it as there and have compassion for yourself (saying those good phrases *May I...* etc. for yourself again). I also add phrases to make the wishes more appropriate, for example, *"May you be happy and be the cause of happiness to others; may you be free from suffering and free others from their suffering"* and so on – sometimes through gritted teeth!

6. Starting with the words *'May we all be..."* we wish all five people together good things with the same phrases – reminding ourselves that we are all human and we all need and deserve compassion and loving kindness.

7. Finally, we widen our good wishes to everyone in the world, all beings on earth, everything in the universe. We widen loving kindness beyond all boundaries, beyond ourselves, and beyond all we know.

Why does this work? Why do I do this?

In practical terms, it has changed my approach to activism as well as life in general.

When dealing with difficult situations, it can be a little annoying, because the practice of Loving Kindness gives me insight and compassion for my opponents! It may not change my words, but it changes the tone, and I feel less anger and adrenalin in me, which is good for my health and well-being. I must be clear that I am no advanced practitioner; you will not observe me showing loving kindness or restraint in every single encounter! Nevertheless, I have observed increasingly the following:

1. If I am listening to someone else's pain, I am more able to listen with compassion without bringing in my own pain – or at least I can see where their pain ends and mine begins. My tension lessens as I have compassion for myself and the suffering person/ people I am with.

2. If I am triggered and I flare up in anger, I am more compassionate for myself rather than feeling guilty – guilt sets off all kinds of emotional turmoil. When I am compassionate for myself, I see what triggered it (e.g. it was the end of the day, and someone said or did the wrong thing and I was too tired and worn out to stop myself reacting). I can also see another human being doing their best who is perhaps tired and at the end of their day. This means I am more likely to apologise – because an apology restores connection.

3. I am more likely than not to separate the words and actions that irritate me from the person. This means, for instance, the recognition that I may fundamentally disagree with the CEO of Leeds Teaching Hospitals on his response to my letter, but I recognise that he is a human being like me, trying to run a complex organisation. I may think the Head of Midwifery is out of order, but she is also a human being under pressure, maybe without the support she needs. I do find this consequence of regular Loving Kindness irritating because I cannot cast people as simply 'the

baddie' anymore! I can now see the human being behind the opponent. When this happens, your attitude and your tone changes. Winning the game is not about beating your opponent; it is getting a version of what you want.

4. If I am practising Loving Kindness regularly and then immediately prior to walking into a difficult conversation or meeting, my attitude changes – towards myself, towards the other(s) and towards the encounter itself. I will often do the practice for everyone who will be in the room, a particularly difficult person, and myself. Then when I walk into the room, I feel calmer, more open and willing to listen – more open to these other human beings in the room, more aware of the baggage they and I bring into this conversation. The conversation may still be tough – I may, for instance, have to be clear about my boundaries and views – but it is delivered with the inner understanding that this might be difficult for the other person too, so my tone softens. I may feel pretty rough after the meeting or encounter, but I feel something else too: a sense of calm, that the world is bigger than this one meeting and the people in it. And I feel kindness and compassion towards everyone who was there – which is why opponents might be surprised to receive an email or card thanking them for their positive contribution to a tough meeting!

Please note, this is no magic bullet for specific conflict resolution or difficult feelings towards others. It is rather a practice that shifts the central paradigm of your life towards kindness and compassion which then begins to reframe

your approach to these situations. To learn more, read
Pema Chödrön's book, *The Places That Scare You*[61].

Tonglen

Thich Nhat Hanh said:

> *"Someone asked me, 'Aren't you worried about the
> state of the world?' I allowed myself to breathe and
> then I said, 'What is most important is not to allow
> your anxiety about what happens in the world to fill
> your heart. If your heart is filled with anxiety, you
> will get sick, and you will not be able to help."* [62]

Tara Brach talks about our human tendency to either
withdraw and shut down, or become overwhelmed and
sink in despair when faced by suffering and intractable
situations. Tonglen, alongside the Loving Kindness Practice,
enables us to turn towards the suffering of others, and our
uncomfortable reactions to it, but then transform these
difficult issues into compassion and loving kindness for all.
It is said to be an advanced practice but I think it is essential
for staying connected to others without making yourself ill.

Tonglen is the Tibetan form of what old Christian
evangelicals might call "Take it to the Lord in prayer," or
as good Catholic friends might say, "Offering it up for the
suffering souls". There are several forms – some for walking
down the street and watching the news, some for a quiet
time of reflection. In the practice, we bring our suffering
selves, our suffering world, our fearfulness and the fear
in our neighbours, we bring them all, all of them as we
breathe in. And as we breathe out, they are transformed

into love and light and compassion, falling gently on a world, desperate and parched. Just as we have the rain cycle – gathering water from the ocean to fall on the hills giving water and life until it returns to the ocean – so we have the love cycle: when all human experience is gathered up, it is transformed into love and compassion, which falls gently on us all, giving us life and flowing through our communities, bringing joy and healing.

My favourite version of Tonglen is a visualisation called 'The Golden Light of Universal Compassion'[63]. I learnt it from Choden, a Tibetan Buddhist Monk and a co-founder of the Mindfulness Association. His practice can be found on YouTube[64]. This is my version of it:

> *First let us find that still point in the storm of our lives. And breathe. Breath in the fresh air and gentle breeze and be still… be still, breathe and be still. Breath in, breath out. Be still.*
>
> *Now imagine the big blue open sky, broad and spacious.*
>
> *And in that sky is a golden gate.*
>
> *Imagine now that gate is opening…*
>
> *And, as you breath out, everything that you hold within you streams out of you towards the golden gate.*
>
> *And as you breath out all your suffering, your pain streams out of you towards the heavenly gate.*
>
> *You breathe out again and your difficult and negative feelings are drawn out of you, towards and through the open gate.*

As you breathe out, you watch as painful memories are drawn out of you and through the golden gate.

As the stream of suffering continues to flow out from you through the golden gate, you can see it go through the gate returning transformed into the light of compassion.

Suffering, pain, difficult memories and feelings pass through the golden gate and are transformed into the light of compassion which falls to Earth as a nourishing rain of love and healing.

We continue to breath in, the suffering of our friends and family are drawn through us to the golden gate, flowing out as love and compassion.

And finally, the suffering of all those we read of and hear of in the news of our country and the world. All the suffering we struggle to watch, all the pain we turn away from, all the people we walk by…

Allow their suffering to flow through you, up through the golden gate, seeing it transform into streams of loving kindness.

Imagine those streams of loving kindness now becoming rivers of love flowing to the difficult places in the world, the homes of the bereaved, the refugee camps, the prisons and torture chambers, the crying children, the grieving mothers, the desperate people in their dinghies.

Let love keep flowing and imagine our world wrapped in bands of white light, the energy of love flowing and bringing healing where it flows…

And finally, see that light flow into you and fill every part of you, every cell in your body, every thought and feeling, filling all the dark places and every part of you with light.

Filled with light, just sit, peacefully, tranquil, content.

The gate in the sky closes, and slowly fades from sight. But we continue to rest in peace and stillness.

The room comes back into focus, the place where we are sat, our feet on the ground, the sounds around us. We breath.

Filled with light, we sit peaceful, content, knowing that we take this light with us wherever we go today, this week, and on.

In your own time, open your eyes and move your body for comfort.

When we are able to turn towards suffering, allowing it to flow through us, enabling it to be transformed into compassion and love, then our capacity to meet suffering without turning away or hardening against it expands exponentially. This truly is going beyond cynicism, to live in Loving Kindness.

To Conclude

Being an activist does not involve anything other than being human. It is about not letting the suffering in the world harden us, but about turning towards suffering and letting it soften us. It is about offering up the suffering of souls and allowing it to be transformed into Love and Compassion and setting it free in ourselves and the world. It is not a magic bullet to resolve each difficult situation; rather, practise shifts the central paradigm of our lives to one of compassion which then begins to reframe our approach to these situations.

Why do I talk about these spiritual matters in the midst of a book on activism? It is because if we are to face and counter suffering and injustice without becoming hard and cynical or overwhelmed and in despair, we have to find something in ourselves that can be both terribly tough but also deeply loving and tender. If we are going to be able to both weep with the victims and talk with compassion to the perpetrators, we are going to need to find a powerful strength within ourselves.

Along with many long-term activists, I have found this strength coming through deep spiritual practice. It can be a matter of embarrassment to discuss such spiritual matters in the midst of discussing maternity care and policy (with good reason), and yet to humanise the system, it is probably necessary.

At a conference I chaired, Michel Odent spoke, starting from the word 'joy'. Joy with Love is the hormone of birth – oxytocin. He asserted that if we have maternity care policies that promote joy, then we will facilitate physiological birth and have care that meets the needs of the mother and baby. A simple spiritual virtue cuts through mind-numbing policy detail to the essence of our practice. Love is the way, whichever way you want to cut the cake. We who wish to make birth a joy, act with love, in love, and are healed by love. It is the only way. And practise makes perfect, and practice makes policy.

Conclusion

～

Changing the Way the Wind Blows

WE MUST START WHERE we began, with a woman giving birth and a midwife whose professional autonomy is compromised. We go back to a young mother taking her first steps in maternity activism, speaking out on injustice, accountability and seeking change.

This book is about how to be an activist. I have talked about the process of being 'woken up' by a series of life events that alerted me to structural injustice in the maternity system – that is a system that should be about health and well-being, causing harm to the mothers and babies it is supposed to care for.

Along with many historians, I see it rooted in the historical socio-economic position of women, whose legacy has not yet been totally acknowledged and overturned in maternity care.

We then moved on to the life of an activist, which as you will observe is not what pays the bills. Like so many other activists, I work to earn money and spend time looking after my family, as well as being active, with all that means in terms of one backside riding three horses. What I hope you can also observe from my book, is that there are many forms of activism, from the classic protest, to writing letters, running support (also read 'empowerment') groups, sitting on committees, running businesses to provide products and services not otherwise available, providing cover and opportunities for others, babysitting, making tea and cake, and generally enabling others to be active, providing friendship, support and love to your sisters and siblings. Activism (and all the other names you can use for it) is a way of life, a way of showing love and compassion for your fellow beings, and within it, there are many roles.

When maternity care harms rather than nurtures women, pregnant people and midwives, then we are complicit if we remain silent. In these pages, you have found many strategies and tactics to hold the system and its leaders to account. It can be scary and challenging, but activism can also be fun.

Where possible, use wit and a light touch; try to make allies rather than enemies, use opponents' own beliefs to leverage in change. But when push comes to shove and there is conflict or an unexpected success, stay focused, stay calm, step back mentally to see what is REALLY going on in the froth and the noise, and then move strategically to make the best of your situation.

And remember, that however personal it feels, this is not about you and your personal success or failure: we act on a vast, historical stage of mother/baby human rights and we are simply doing our little bit for change, whether it is successful or not.

The activist life has a high rate of attrition through burnout and breakdown, especially for women and certainly in maternity. This is difficult to talk about both on a personal and a systemic level, but it needs to be acknowledged. For instance, in maternity we ask mothers of young families, whilst also raising their families and often working for their living, to represent their peers *unpaid*. This is preposterous, and demonstrates the structural discrimination against women and mothers still endemic in the system.

We can do what we can to avoid breakdown and burnout but we cannot always avoid it. And so as with the other side of activism, there are strategies and wisdom that we can use to nurture and heal ourselves through this dark time. Coming out the other side, we may be wounded but we have strength and resilience: it is not a question of whether we are activists, but **how** we are activists.

And we have our allies! Our tribe of family and friends, our colleagues across professional, social, political and cultural boundaries – even our opponents. We work with those who will work with us for the benefit of mothers and babies, and ultimately families and communities. In our allies, we can find friendship and laughter, support and a shoulder to cry on, wisdom, knowledge, backup. With our allies, we can find a role that suits our personality and circumstances.

TOGETHER WE CAN DO THIS!

Political activist and theologian Jim Wallis said that politicians of all kinds are "wet-fingered".

> *"You can't change a nation by replacing one wet-fingered politician with another. You change a nation when you change the wind. You change the way the wind is blowing."*[65]

We do not seek to change one wet-fingered politician for another, but what we need to do is 'change the way the wind is blowing'. As with women's suffrage, generations of women, mothers, midwives and their supporters – of all political colours – will need to act to make humane maternity care 'the way the wind blows' . . .

And I am looking at **YOU**.

So can you write a letter? Hold a candle in a vigil?
Can you organise a protest? Lead a chant, sing a song?
Will you stand in solidarity?
Give tea and sympathy,
Have her back when your sibling is set upon?
'What can I contribute?' is the question that we ask you to ask.
Availability not ability is the question.
We must organise and unionise
We must claim our democratic right
The battle must be fought to be won.

Sisters,

We need to be determined, clever, fun.

We need to band together to organise and unionise, to write letters and demonstrate.

And we need to educate, educate, educate.

Talk to our daughters, sisters, mothers;

Talk to our sons, husbands, brothers;

And we need to fearlessly claim our heritage to birth and bring to birth,

To be the women, the mothers, the midwives we are.

We need to campaign as determinedly and creatively as we give birth,

Because our daughters are worth it

– and so are we.

Glossary

ACOG

American College of Obstetricians and Gynaecologists

AIMS

Association for the Improvement of Maternity Services

ARM

Association of Radical Midwives

ASQUAM

Achieving Sustainable Quality in Maternity Services

A one-day, all stakeholders event to identify easy-to-implement changes to service that would have positive benefits. It used to be held bi-annually at the Bradford Royal Infirmary.

BBA

Born Before Arrival. The acronym for babies that arrive before the midwife or emergency services get there. It can also apply to babies who are born before the parent makes it to hospital!

Cochrane Review

A Cochrane Review is "a systematic review that attempts to identify, appraise and synthesize all the evidence that meets pre-specified eligibility criteria to answer a research question. Researchers use explicit, systematic methods aimed at minimizing bias, to produce more reliable findings to inform decision-making. Cochrane Reviews may be updated to reflect the findings of new evidence because the results can change the conclusions of a review. They are therefore valuable sources of information for those receiving and providing care, as well as for decision-makers and researchers." www.cochranelibrary.com/about/about-cochrane-reviews

EPAU

Early Pregnancy Assessment Unit

FOI requests

Freedom of Information requests

IM/IMs

Independent midwife/independent midwives. These midwives usually, but not always, operate outside the NHS, although they must still register with the NMC (Nursing

---

and Midwifery Council) to work. They are commissioned and paid for by the parents and families themselves.

MLU

Midwifery-Led Unit, often also called a Birth Centre. It is a maternity unit where midwives are the lead healthcare professionals (HCPs): there are no doctors/obstetricians. You have to be transferred to an obstetric unit if you require a doctor.

Moral Injury

Psychiatrist Jonathan Shay coined the term "moral injury" as a "betrayal of what is right by someone who holds legitimate authority in a high stakes situation." The definition of moral injury has since been expanded to include "perpetrating, failing to prevent, bearing witness to acts that ultimately transgress one's deeply held moral beliefs," creating dissonance.

MSLC

Maternity Services Liaison Committee – the once statutory stakeholder committee overseeing maternity services in a hospital or area. The statutory requirement was removed whilst I was in post as Chair and eventually it was replaced by MVP, which was in turn replaced by MNVP. Ideally, it would be chaired by a layperson.

MVP

Maternity Voices Partnership, the stakeholder committee that replaced MSLCs and has now been replaced again by MNVPs (see next item).

MNVP

Maternity & Neonatal Voices Partnerships (to make sure we have another mouthful)! This is not a statutory body, although it is good practice and policy to have one. In the past, this was chaired by a layperson like myself, but less so now. Follow AIMS campaign work to learn more.

NM

Neighbourhood Midwives. This was a group of midwives who set up a midwifery partnership. They wanted to be an autonomous professional body outside the secondary care-based maternity system of the current NHS structures described in this book, but contracted into the NHS to deliver a continuity of carer service, offering the local health commissioners the excellent outcomes such teams deliver.

PPH

Postpartum Haemorrhage

RCM

Royal College of Midwives

RCOG

Royal College of Obstetricians and Gynaecologists

VBAC

Vaginal Birth After Caesarean

References

Foreword

[1] Savage, W (2008) Margie Polden Memorial Lecture: 'Maternity Matters: can the Government deliver?' *Journal of the Association of Chartered Physiotherapists in Women's Health*, Spring 2009, 104, 5–11

[2] *Listen to Mums: Ending the Postcode Lottery on Perinatal Care*, Parliamentary Report on Birth Trauma, Theo Clarke MP, May 2024, www.theo-clarke.org.uk/birth-trauma-report

A Note About Language

[3] en.wikipedia.org/wiki/Global_majority

Introduction

[4] Marjorie Tew, *Safer Childbirth?: A Critical History of Maternity Care*; Free Association Books; Third Edition 1998. This is a classic book and **everyone** should read it. **EVERYONE.**

See *Further Reading* for other histories and critiques of the socio-economic history of maternity.

Making Change Happen: Disrupting the Patterns

[5] A D&C – or dilation and curettage – is a surgical procedure where the cervix is dilated or expanded so that the uterine lining can be scraped with a curette (a spoon-shaped instrument) to remove products or tissue.

[6] Jim Wallis, *God's Politics: Why the American Right Gets It Wrong and the Left Doesn't Get It*, Lion Books, 2005, p22. *"You change society by changing the wind. Change the wind, transform the debate, recast the discussion, alter the context in which political discussions are being made, and you will change the outcomes… You will be surprised at how fast the politicians adjust to the change in the wind."*

Part 1: Birth of an Activist

Chapter 1: The Wake-up Call

[7] Here is one of the many articles I would have come across. Jean Robinson, 'Post Traumatic Stress Disorder', ISSN 0256-5004 (Print) *AIMS Journal*, 2007, Vol 19, No 1

[8] 'Healthcare's compassion crisis', Stephen Trxeciak (2018) TED Talk. Available at: www.ted.com/talks/stephen_trzeciak_healthcare_s_compassion_crisis_jan_2018

Octavia Wiseman, 'Selfless Angel or Selfish Cow: How we judge women's choices around motherhood', *Essentially Midirs*; Jan 2013; www.researchgate.net/publication/302249856_Selfless_angel_or_selfish_cow_How_we_judge_women's_choices_around_motherhood

'Why aren't we more compassionate?' Daniel Goldman (2007) TED Talk. Available at www.ted.com/talks/daniel_goleman_why_aren_t_we_more_compassionate

See *Further Reading* for more references on the subject of kindness in the health service.

Chapter 3: The Game Changer

[9] Michael Odent, *Birth and Breastfeeding, Rediscovering the needs of women during pregnancy and childbirth*, Clairview Books, 2003 – see *Notes on References* section.

Madlen Davies for MailOnline and Sophie Borland, Health Correspondent, 'The secret to a quick, painless childbirth? Just don't think about it and ban your partner from the room, leading doctor claims', *The Daily Mail*, July 2015, www.dailymail.co.uk/health/article-3147111/The-secret-quick-painless-childbirth-Just-don-t-think-ban-partner-room-leading-doctor-claims.html

[10] waitforwhite.com/

For example; 'Infant Mental Health Week: The importance of Delayed Cord Clamping (DCC) and its impact on brain development', The Royal College of Midwives, 10th June 2016, waitforwhite.com/published-articles

[11] PPH – See reference 15.

Chapter 4: Building My Vision for Birth and Finding Independent Midwifery

[12] The references in the policy came from the Cochrane Review – see *Glossary* for description. You can find the latest Cochrane Review of water birth here.

There is also a link to the historical reviews including the 1997 and 2002 reviews relevant to this story.

Elizabeth R Cluett, Ethel Burns, Anna Cuthbert; 'Immersion in water during labour and birth', Version published: 16 May 2018, www.cochranelibrary.com/cdsr/doi/10.1002/14651858. CD000111.pub4/full?highlightAbstract=waterbirth

[13] Choices newsletter. Subscribe at choices@aquabirths.co.uk

[14] *Desperate Midwives*: The Open University and BBC, Copyright © Open University, www.open.ac.uk/about/main/management/policies-and-statements/copyright-ou-websites, The Open University, 2015, directed by Josh Whitehead

[15] Neither myself nor my colleague Michelle Irving can remember/have a record of the studies quoted back then. However, we can both find studies going back to the 1980s whose results show that parity (the number of previous live births) is not associated with PPH, certainly in high-income settings. There are a selection of studies here: www.midwifery.org.uk/articles/grand-multiparity-and-pph-risk

The latest studies have no association between parity and PPH, for example:

obgyn.onlinelibrary.wiley.com/doi/10.1111/aogs.12950, 2016

pmc.ncbi.nlm.nih.gov/articles/PMC10874836, 2024

[16] www.homebirth.org.uk/marycronk See *Notes on References* section for more of what Mark Cronk says.

[17] www.thelancet.com/series/midwifery

[18] Sandall J, Fernandez Turienzo C, Devane D, Soltani H, Gillespie P, Gates S, Jones LV, Shennan AH, Rayment-Jones H. 'Midwife continuity of care models versus other models of care for childbearing women'. *Cochrane Database of Systematic Reviews*, 2024, Issue 4. Art. No.: CD004667. DOI: 10.1002/14651858.CD004667.pub6. www.cochrane.org/CD004667/PREG_are-midwife-continuity-care-models-versus-other-models-care-childbearing-women-better-women-and-their-babies See *Notes on References* section/

[19] Emma Ashworth, 'The Consequences of Discontinuing Continuity', *AIMS Journal*, 2018, Vol 30, No1 www.aims.org.uk/journal/item/discontinuing-continuity

Part 2: Being a Birth Activist

Chapter 5: Vision into Action

[20] S Pokhrel, M A Quigley, J Fox-Rushby, F McCormick, A Williams, P Trueman, R Dodds, M J Renfrew, 'Potential economic impacts from improving breastfeeding rates in the UK', 2014, adc.bmj.com/content/archdischild/100/4/334.full.pdf

[21] 'Life Cycle Assessment of Disposable and Reusable Nappies in the UK', 2005, assets.publishing.service.gov.uk/media/5a7c4096ed915d7d70d1d993/scho0505bjcw-e-e.pdf

'Life Cycle Analysis of Nappies/Absorbent Hygiene Products 2021/23 - EV0493' 2023. randd.defra.gov.uk/ProjectDetails?ProjectId=20622

[22] Two blogs which summarise the reports' history over the last 20 years:

www.thenappylady.co.uk/news/revised-cloth-nappy-lifecycle-report-2008.html

www.thenappylady.co.uk/news/life-cycle-assessment-of-disposable-and-reusable-nappies-in-the-uk-2023.html

[23] Birthplace Cohort Study: www.npeu.ox.ac.uk/birthplace/results

'Perinatal and maternal outcomes by planned place of birth for healthy women with low risk pregnancies: the Birthplace in England national prospective cohort study', 2011, www.bmj.com/content/343/bmj.d7400

[24] D. Hughes, M. Kirkham and R. Deery, *Tensions and Barriers in Improving Maternity Care: The Story of a Birth Centre*, Routledge, June 2010.

D. Hughes, M. Kirkham and R. Deery, 'Why birth centres fail', *AIMS Journal*: Volume 24, No. 2, 2012–13 www.aims.org.uk/journal/item/why-birth-centres-fail

[25] Borninbradford.nhs.uk

[26] Victoria Finan, 'Bradford stillbirth and perinatal deaths highest in the region as charity leader calls for inquiry', *The Yorkshire Post*, February 2022, www.yorkshirepost.co.uk/health/bradford-stillbirth-and-perinatal-deaths-highest-in-the-region-3574513

Chapter 6: Holding to Account

[27] National Maternity Review: Better Care: Improving outcomes of maternity services in England. A Five Year ForwardView for maternity care', www.england.nhs.uk/wp-content/uploads/2016/02/national-maternity-review-report.pdf

[28] D. Hughes, M. Kirkham and R. Deery, *Tensions and Barriers in Improving Maternity Care: The Story of a Birth Centre*, Routledge, June 2010.

Chapter 7: Media Skills for the Campaigner

[29] "I had to pay for my home birth", 2007, *BBC News*, news.bbc.co.uk/1/hi/health/6519017.stm

Chapter 8: Finding your Allies

[30] Birthplace Cohort Study: www.npeu.ox.ac.uk/birthplace/results

Part 3: Activist Reborn

Chapter 10: The Death of an Activist: Burnout

[31] www.mindfulnessassociation.net/free-resources/free-daily-online-mindfulness-meditation See *Useful Organisations.*

[32] Dr Gavin Francis, *Recovery: The Lost Art of Convalescence*, Profile Books, Wellcome Collection, 2022

[33] *Woman's Hour* series on Menopause www.bbc.co.uk/programmes/p05tpw79

[34] *28ish Days Later* on Radio 4
www.bbc.co.uk/sounds/brand/p0bvg9nm

[35] Dr Jade Teta, *Metabolic Renewal: Restore, Re-balance, Results* can only be purchased with the program online at www.metabolic.com/products/metabolic-renewal-digital

[36] Tara Brach, *Radical Acceptance: Embracing Your Life With the Heart of a Buddha*, Random House, 2004. This book is an international classic and is the book that helped me pick up the pieces and put myself back together. I recommend it wholeheartedly.

[37] Katherine May, *Wintering*, Penguin, 2020

[38] Caroline Criado-Perez, *Invisible Women*, Vintage, 2020

[39] The concept of safe childbirth. 'Refusal of Medically Recommended Treatment During Pregnancy', 2016
www.acog.org/clinical/clinical-guidance/committee-opinion/articles/2016/06/refusal-of-medically-recommended-treatment-during-pregnancy

Nadine Pilley Edwards, *Birthing Autonomy: Women's Experiences of Planning Home Births*, Routledge, 2005. Nadine's book studies in-depth the reasons women make the choices they do.

Chapter 11: Born Again: Activism beyond Cynicism

[40] The Ockenden Report by Donna Ockenden, Chair of the Independent Maternity Review, March 2022, www.gov.uk/government/publications/final-report-of-the-ockenden-review

See *Notes on References* section for the background to the Ockenden Report.

[41] The Report of the Morecambe Bay Investigation: https://assets.publishing.service.gov.uk/media/5a7f3d7240f0b62305b85efb/47487_MBI_Accessible_v0.1.pdf
See *Notes on References* section

[42] Jonathan Freedland, *The Escape Artist*, John Murray Press, 2022

[43] Liberation and contextual theologies books

Leonardo Boff, Clodovis Boff et al, *Introducing Liberation Theology*, Burns and Oats, 1987. This book has never been bettered. I dare anyone to read the story that is the first chapter of this little book without a lump in the throat: it is a breastfeeding woman that converts Clodovis Boff to this path

Pablo Galdamez; *Faith of a People: The Life of a Basic Christian Community in El Salvador*; Orbis/Dove/CIIR London 1986. A book that also expresses this theology in practical and story form.

[44] Exodus 1:15-20 NIV

[45] Mark 7: 24-29 NIV

[46] Moral Injury: see *Glossary* for description. See *Further Reading* for more on moral injury/distress.

[47] National Maternity Review: Better Care: Improving outcomes of maternity services in England. A Five Year Forward View for maternity care', www.england.nhs.uk/wp-content/uploads/2016/02/national-maternity-review-report.pdf

[48] 'IMs and insurance', ISSN 0256-5004 (Print), *AIMS Journal*, 2017, Vol 29 No 1 www.aims.org.uk/journal/item/ims-and-insurance

[49] *Listen to Mums: Ending the Postcode Lottery on Perinatal Care*, Parliamentary Report on Birth Trauma, Theo Clarke MP, May 2024, www.theo-clarke.org.uk/birth-trauma-report

[50] 'Saving Lives Improving Mothers' Care 2024: Key messages Lay Summary', MBRRACE-UK_Maternal_Report_2024_Lay_Summary_V1.0.pdf

[51] March with Midwives: A grassroots organisation led by mothers, doulas and birth workers: www.facebook.com/marchwithmidwives/

[52] Pregnant Then Screwed: pregnantthenscrewed.com/ See *Useful Organisations*.

[53] Birthrights: birthrights.org.uk/ See *Useful Organisations*.

[54] Maya Angelou, *Wouldn't Take Nothing for my Journey Now*, Virago, 1995

55 Mark Williams, John Teasdale, Zindel Segal and Jon Kabat-Zinn, *he Mindful Way Through Depression: Freeing Yourself from Chronic Unhappiness*, Guilford Press, 2007, (page 163). See *Notes on References* section.

56 Tara Brach, *Radical Acceptance: Embracing Your Life With the Heart of a Buddha*, Random House, 2004, 'Tea with Mara', pp 75-6

57 Tara Brach, *True Refuge: Finding Peace And Freedom In Your Own Awakened Heart*, Hay House, 2013. RAIN practice: Chapter 5, p 65

58 Bishop Michael Curry, Royal Wedding Sermon, 20th May 2018, www.npr.org/sections/thetwo-way/2018/ 05/20/6127 98691/bishop-michael-currys-royal-wedding-sermon-full-text-of-the-power-of-love

59 Thich Nhat Hạnh, *The Art of Living*, Random House, 2022 (pp 18-20)

60 Philip Yancey, *What's So Amazing About Grace?*, Zondervan Publishing House, 1997

61 Pema Chödrön, *The Places that Scare You*, Shambhala, 2007. Her classic book is a good place to start reading and has a very good description of the full Loving Kindness practice.

62 Thich Nhất Hạnh, Facebook post, 10th October 2016, www. facebook.com/thichnhathanh/posts/10154203709544635

63 Akong Tulku Rinpoche, *Taming the Tiger; Tibetan Teachings on Right Conduct, Mindfulness, and Universal*

Compassion, Inner Traditions International, 1995. It is from this text that Choden shares the Golden Gate Practice.

[64] The Golden Light of Universal Compassion, Choden's Tonglen practice on YouTube taken from *Taming the Tiger*, www.youtube.com/watch?v=scXWOpCcQKg

How to be an Activist

Conclusion: Changing the Way the Wind Blows

[65] Jim Wallis in his speech to the Faith in Politics conference, 29th March 2001. See reference 6.

Notes on References

Chapter 3, reference 9

Michel Odent on privacy: *"To give birth to her baby, the mother needs privacy. She needs to feel unobserved. The newborn baby needs the skin of the mother, the smell of the mother, her breast. These are all needs that we hold in common with the other mammals, but which humans have learned to neglect, to ignore or even deny."*

Chapter 4, reference 16

Mary Cronk: *The Midwife: A Professional Servant Chapter 4, The Midwife Mother Relationship*, Ed. Mavis Kirkham, Palgrave Macmillan, 2010

"Mary Cronk explores the concept that a midwife is a professional servant, employed by the woman (either directly or indirectly) to care for her. Mary asks us to remember that anyone providing a service is a servant, that a midwife has a profession, and that therefore a midwife is a professional servant, like it or not. Mary challenges midwives to free themselves of the notion

that they have power over those they care for, to stop 'letting'
and 'allowing' because she explains that a midwife has no right
to 'presume a power' or to 'use that power to control women."
www.aims.org.uk/journal/item/book-reviews-22-3#2

Chapter 4, reference 18

Continuity of Carer: AIMS has loads of information on
this topic and updates regularly on the latest research and
policy: aims-position-paper-continuity-of-carer.pdf

www.aims.org.uk/campaigning/item/implementing-coc –
a list of key milestones and resources.

Chapter 11, reference 40

Background information on the events leading to the
Ockenden Report, with thanks to Gill George, a leading
campaigner, for co-producing this information. The
midwife perspective is missing and would change some of
the summary below, but because of what happened to those
who spoke up, I did not feel able to involve them.

This was a review/report into baby deaths at the Shrewsbury
and Telford Hospital Trust over a 20-year period, and
arose after concerns were raised in a number of quarters
and in particular by parents whose babies had died or been
profoundly harmed. Remember that baby deaths are the
tip of the iceberg in terms of quality of care – the issues
raised in the report would be experienced within the whole
population, not just those who lost their babies.

A common thread in so many stories from Shropshire's
troubled maternity service is that women were not

listened to. Their needs and the needs of their babies were disregarded. From autumn 2016 onwards, the Trust began repeated short-notice temporary closures of the three rural maternity units in Shropshire. The attacks on the rural MLUs led to three magnificent coordinated campaigns in the towns of Ludlow, Bridgnorth and Oswestry. These were led by local mothers, supported by a local NHS defence campaign, and attracted overwhelming support from the local communities.

The testimonials posted on their Facebook groups make sobering reading of the contrast in care between the MLUs and the Obstetric Unit. Family and public views were disregarded by the Trust and by Shropshire maternity commissioners when the three rural units were closed. This left families forced to drive long distances during labour or if there were concerns pre or postnatal. The Trust has been very cagey about its 'Births Before Arrival' figures.

Meanwhile, midwives faced compulsory transfer from rural MLUs to the very different environment of the Obstetric Unit in Telford. This – together with the emerging story of avoidable baby deaths at Shrewsbury and Telford Hospital Trust – resulted in an exodus of skilled midwives. Subsequently, staff shortages led to routine closures of the last remaining MLU, the 'Alongside MLU' at Telford. Home births have always been discouraged. Maternal choice isn't high up the agenda in Shropshire despite the Better Births Report recommendations. We understand four midwives tried to raise concerns about what was happening in maternity services; they were all silenced one way or another and left the Trust.

The parallel story is the 'drip drip drip' of avoidable harm and deaths in Shropshire's maternity services, and the brave fight for justice by bereaved parents in the area. Two couples in particular stand out as heroes. Without their relentless and years-long fight, the Ockenden Report would not have happened.

It is clear now that hospital leaders and leaders in the wider NHS had known of overwhelming safety concerns for many years. They chose to look the other way. That much is clear from several sources, including old Board papers. Was there a systematic cover up that took place while babies and women continued to die? That has not been excluded. And in that 20-year period, poor care led to the deaths of more than 200 babies.

Chapter 11, reference 41

The Report of the Morecambe Bay Investigation, March 2015, by Dr Bill Kirkup, CBE: *"This Report details a distressing chain of events that began with serious failures of clinical care in the maternity unit at Furness General Hospital, part of what became the University Hospitals of Morecambe Bay NHS Foundation Trust. The result was avoidable harm to mothers and babies, including tragic and unnecessary deaths."* (p5)

Chapter 11, reference 55

This quotation is a good explanation of the thinking behind mindfulness and how our minds work: *"A century ago, Sigmund Freud popularised the idea that we all have an* *unconscious that lies deep below the surface of our awareness, motivating our actions in ways that are highly complex and that take considerable time to unearth and understand. Those in mainstream academic psychology rejected such ideas as unprovable and focused instead on observable behaviour (in a movement known as 'behaviourism'). So fierce was the reaction against Freud that it was only in the late 1960s and the 1970s that behaviourally oriented psychotherapists started to take seriously the interior world of their patients: the subjective domain of thoughts, memories, ideas, projections, and plans. And they made a remarkable discovery: most of what drives our emotions and behaviour is not deeply unconscious, but just below the surface of our awareness. Not only that, but this rich interior world, with its motivations, expectations, interpretations, and story lines, is accessible to all of us if we dare to look. We can all become more aware of the 'stream of consciousness' going on in our minds, moment by moment. It often takes the form a running commentary. If it is potentially damaging to us, it is not because it is buried deep in the psyche but because it is left virtually unattended. **We have gotten so used to its whisperings that we don't even notice it is here. And so, it shapes our lives.** "*

Further Reading

Other histories and critiques of the socio-economic history and culture of maternity

Donnison, J., *Midwives and Medical Men: a History of the Struggle for the Control of Childbirth*, Routledge; Second Edition, 1988

Ehrenreich, B., English, D., *Witches, Midwives and Nurses*, Feminist Press, 2010

Fielder, A., *Going Into Labour: Childbirth In Capitalism*, Pluto Press, 2024

Kirkham, M., *The Midwife Mother Relationship*, Palgrave Macmillan 2010

"This covers topics including the effects of emotional labour, poverty and health policy. It brings together classic and current research to establish key tenets for maternity care within hospital and home. It remains a definitive guide to the complex area of midwife-mother relations" (www.aims.org.uk/journal/item/book-reviews-22-3#2).

Murphy-Lawless, J., *Reading Birth and Death: A History of Obstetric Thinking*, Cork University Press 1998

Odent, Dr Michel, *Do We Need Midwives?* Pinter & Martin Ltd, 2015

In addition to the histories cited above, this article gives an analysis of the invidious position women and midwives find themselves:

Wiseman, O., 'Selfless Angel or Selfish Cow: How we judge women's choices around motherhood', *Essentially Midirs*; Jan 2013; www.researchgate.net/publication/302249856_Selfless_angel_or_selfish_cow_How_we_judge_women's_choices_around_motherhood

Wallis, J., *The Soul of Politics: A Practical and Prophetic Vision for Change*, HarperCollins, 1995
Jim Wallis marries Christian morality US-style to Christian social justice and peace teachings, challenging the polarities of much political and faith-based debate (for instance, on abortion) and offering practical justice-based political solutions to current societal problems. I am told senior figures in the New Labour Government read his book. His challenge is still relevant today.

Other links to Kindness in the Health Service

My thanks goes to Midwife and Professional Midwife Advocate Tracy Curran for this list.

Byrom, S. and Downe, S., *The Roar Behind the Silence: Why kindness, compassion and respect matter in maternity care*, Pinter & Martin, 2015

Fryburg, D., (2022) 'Kindness as a stress reduction-health promotion intervention: A review of the psychology of caring.' *American Journal of Lifestyle Medicine*. 16(1) pp. 89-100.457.

Fryburg, D. (2023) 'Kindness isn't just about being nice: The value proposition of kindness as viewed through the lens of incivility in the healthcare workplace.' *Behavioral Sciences*. 13(6)

Mathers, N. (2016) 'Compassion and the science of kindness: Harvard Davis Lecture 2015.' *British Journal of General Practice*. 66(648) 525-527.

Unwin, J. (2018). 'Kindness, emotions and human relationships: The blind spot in public policy'. Carnegie UK. Available online at: carnegieuktrust.org.uk/publications/kindness-emotions-and-human-relationships-the-blind-spot-in-public-policy/

West, M., *Compassionate leadership*, Swirling Leaf Press, 2021

West, M., Bailey, S. & Williams, E., (2020), 'The courage of compassion'. London: The Kings Fund. Available online at: www.kingsfund.org.uk/insight-and-analysis/reports/courage-compassion-supporting-nurses-midwives

Hunter, B., Henley, J., Fenwick, J., et al. (2018). 'Work, health and emotional lives of midwives in the United Kingdom: The UK WHELM study'. Cardiff: School of Healthcare Sciences, Cardiff University

Hunter, B., Fenwick, J., Sidebotham, M., & Henley, J., 'Midwives in the United Kingdom: Levels of burnout, depression, anxiety and stress and associated predictors', PMID: 31473405 DOI: 10.1016/j.midw.2019.08.008

Key conclusions and implications for practice: Many UK midwives are experiencing high levels of stress, burnout, anxiety and depression, which should be of serious concern to the profession and its leaders. NHS-employed clinical midwives are at much greater risk of emotional distress than others surveyed, which has serious implications for the delivery of high-quality, safe maternity care. It is also of serious concern that younger, more recently qualified midwives recorded some of the highest burnout, stress, anxiety and depression scores, as did midwives who self-reported a disability. There is considerable scope for change across the service. Proactive support needs to be offered to younger, recently qualified midwives and midwives with a disability to help sustain their emotional well-being. The profession needs to lobby for systems-level changes in how UK maternity care is resourced and provided. Making this happen will require support and commitment from a range of relevant stakeholders, at regional and national levels.

On Moral Distress/Moral Injury

Once again, my thanks go to Midwife and Professional Midwife Advocate Tracy Curran in the compilation of this list.

Delima-Tokarz, T., 'The Psychiatric Ramifications of Moral Injury Among Veterans', Published Online: 1 May 2017 doi.org/10.1176/appi.ajp-rj.2016.110505

Fourie, C., (2015) 'Moral distress and moral conflict in clinical ethics', *Bioethics*, 29(2), pp. 91-97.

Jameton, A., *Nursing practice: the ethical issues*, Englewood Cliffs: Prentice-Hall, 1984.

Koening, H., Al Zaben, F., 'Moral Injury: An Increasingly Recognized and Widespread Syndrome,' *Journal of Religious Health*, 2021; 60(5): 2989–3011, published online 2021 Jul 10, doi: 10.1007/s10943-021-01328-0

Lamiani, G., Borghi, L., Argentero, P. (2017) 'When healthcare professionals cannot do the right thing: A systematic review of moral distress and its correlates'. *Journal of Health Psychology*. 22 (1), pp. 51-67.

Litz, B., Stein, N., Delaney, E, Lebowitz, L., Nash, W., Silva, C. & Maguen, S. (2009) 'Moral injury and moral repair in war veterans: A preliminary model and intervention strategy'. *Clinical Psychology Review*. 29(8), pp. 695-706.

O'Connor, A., (2021) 'Moral injury'. *Therapy Today*. 32(2). Pp.34-37.

Shay, J., *Achilles in Vietnam: Combat trauma and the undoing of character*, Scribner, 1995

Smith, J., *Nurturing maternity staff: How to tackle trauma, stress and burnout to create a positive working culture in the NHS.* Pinter & Martin, 2021.

Tessman, L., 'Moral distress in health care: when is it fitting?' *Med Health Care Philos.* 2020 Jun;23(2):165-177. doi: 10.1007/s11019-020-09942-7. PMID: 32034572

Webster, G. & Baylis, F. Moral residue. In S. Rubin, & L. Zoloth (Eds.), *Margin of error: The ethics of mistakes in the practice of medicine.* Hagerstown, MD: University Publishing Group, Inc., 2000

Videos:

'The history of moral injury'. Kings College London. (2021) Available at: www.youtube.com/watch?v=QX8_QkNUoy8

'Understanding moral injury'. Health Education England. (2021) Available at: www.youtube.com/watch?v=AybMP LVbtvg&t=5s

'Handling moral injury'. Health Education England. (2021). Available at: www.youtube.com/watch?v=7XXJ zTy51LM&t=4s

Mindfulness:

Germer, Dr Christopher K., *The Mindful Path to Self-Compassion – Freeing yourself from destructive thoughts and emotions*, Guilford Press 2009. Germer's book is stuffed full of research if this is what you are looking for

Treleaven, David A., *Trauma-Sensitive Mindfulness: Practice for Safe and Transformative Healing*, Norton London 2018. One of the standouts of this book is that Treleaven recognises discrimination and racism as structural elements that overlay trauma experienced by individuals. This is particularly relevant to maternity services and the ongoing systemic discrimination and racism that occurs in it.

Other people to look out for include Kristin Nef, Jon Kabat-Zihn, Rob Nairn, Jack Kornfield, Pema Chödrön, Choden, Thich Naht Hanh and Greg Boyle, who provide research and teaching on compassion and mindfulness from the medical, psychological, Buddhist and even Christian perspectives, as most suits you.

Useful Organisations

This is by no means a comprehensive list of organisations where people can seek support and solidarity. It is simply a sample to start your search for the organisations that suit you.

Association for Improvements in the Maternity Services (AIMS)

www.aims.org.uk/

This is an excellent organisation with one of the most comprehensive open-access websites for parents and professionals alike. They offer information, references and books with up-to-date evidence on such things as induction, the third stage of labour, parental rights, and so on. They do a lot of work on maternity policies and national guidelines, on access to services like home birth and midwifery-led care, and they challenge poor standards of care and coercion of parents. Their database of journal articles is massive and they also have a helpline for parents struggling with their choices and decisions being respected by providers. For example, all the parents I worked with who used their home birth letter got their home birth. This is all done by volunteers on a miniscule budget. Use them, donate to them and volunteer if you can – this organisation is gold!

Association of Radical Midwives (ARM)

www.midwifery.org.uk

In my humble view, this is the midwives' equivalent to AIMS. This is a support organisation for midwives who want to practise traditional with woman midwifery. Over the years, as the need has arisen and continues in various forms to this day, the ARM has run retreats for exhausted midwives to refresh, has set up a research database and journal for midwives and midwifery, peer information exchange, and a support group. ARM campaigns on issues such as midwifery regulation, midwives and women's autonomy, malicious reporting of midwives to the regulator, and much more. They have organised public protests, letter writing campaigns, round-table strategy meetings with stakeholders and much, much more. Their journal is a good read, their conferences and study days are excellent and if you are a member, you have access to their database and their support groups. Notwithstanding the ebb and flow of controversies, if there was no ARM, someone would have to set one up; midwives and the midwifery profession NEED an ARM.

Birthrights

birthrights.org.uk/

This is an excellent organisation – it provides expert legal advice and representation to parents, midwives, doulas and other birth workers. It provides free information on the legal rights of parents around pregnancy and birth, and it runs some excellent campaigns. It provides training to midwives to inform and support them in upholding mother/baby human rights. In the face of structural discrimination that has had up to five times as many Black women dying around childbirth than white women, Birthrights has set out to increase Black and ethnic minority participation and representation in the organisation. I have enormous respect for Birthrights.

La Leche League

laleche.org.uk

and

Association of Breastfeeding Mothers

abm.me.uk/

These two organisations, along with the much-missed Sure Start programmes, were the mainstay of my breastfeeding support and were the places I referred mothers. The practical and research knowledge leaders and even peer supporters possessed was phenomenal, and the skilful facilitation of groups enabled women and people to share experiences and tips that enriched and skilled everyone in breastfeeding but also general parenting skills, birth trauma and future birth choices. These groups can be immensely empowering. I would counsel every pregnant woman or person to find such a group which suits them before they give birth. The helplines have also been lifesavers for many desperate parents – I cannot thank these volunteers enough for their dedication and personal sacrifices.

March with Midwives

www.facebook.com/marchwithmidwives

If you want to do something but you don't know what, join this massive community of activists from all professions and walks of life, because together we can! A place of solidarity, discussion and planning.

Mindfulness Association

www.mindfulnessassociation.net/free-resources/free-daily-online-mindfulness-meditation/

The Mindfulness Association (MA) provide free daily sits, Monday to Friday, 10.30am and 7pm. This is a good place to start a practice because you only have to make the effort to be there and there is a supportive community too. All the leaders are themselves teachers, often with a vast experience from life or their profession. I have learnt much from them. The MA also run courses on Mindfulness and Compassion so if you want to dive deeper, this is a good place to go.

Plum Village

plumvillage.org

The community that grew around Thich Naht Hanh provides free podcasts and articles to support activists to stay grounded. Friends and colleagues heartily recommend it. Here is one example: plumvillage.org/podcast/mindful-activism-from-anxiety-to-agency-episode-57

Pregnant and Screwed

pregnantthenscrewed.com

I came across them on Twitter (now X) whilst tweeting during the pandemic. This dynamic political and media savvy group of angry women and people who demand that the system be changed have been a joy to watch from a distance. What they say: "Join our funny, ferocious crew challenging the systems which oppress us and become a Pregnant Then Screwed member today. We can't do this without you."

Urban Theology Union

utusheffield.org.uk

Rooted in a deprived urban area of Sheffield and Theologies of Liberation, UTU has forged a path of practical radical lived discipleship and theology rooted in the scriptural imperative of God's priority for the poor. UTU challenges people who cross its path to live lives of solidarity in deprived urban areas of the UK, and has founded or enabled a variety of faith communities and vocations to this end along with programmes of study and practice to learn the theological and scriptural basis of radical solidarity based living. Coming to UTU is life-changing – and you always end up poorer because the imperative is solidarity with the poor, the oppressed and the downtrodden – John Vincent called it 'the journey downwards'. This small and agile organisation continues as a members' organisation setting up small study communities, study days, book writing clubs, PhD writing, and so on.

Acknowledgements

THEY SAY IT TAKES A TRIBE to raise a child, but it is also true that it takes a tribe to write and publish a book. And these acknowledgements are a tribute to my tribe.

There are four people who helped me write this book – I asked them to be my mentors and supervisors. Without them, this book would not have been written, and without them, it would not be the book that it is. The Urban Theology Union, where I was trained in practical liberation theology and community organising, have a PhD and book writing club.

A tentative conversation on my part had me joining the group with a passionate and funny pitch and the archive of my years of talks and analysis. The humour, discernment, wisdom and encouragement I received from my three mentors was phenomenal; they persuaded me to write my story rather than simply talking about what needed to change, and so the book you read is in no small part because of them. Thank you, Ian Duffield, Robin Pagan and Rob Hoch-Yidokodilton.

For Ian Duffield, there is a particular acknowledgement, because as one of my tutors in the 1990s, he heard his teaching come back at him in my words. The joint reflection on that teaching and what I did with it is precious wisdom, only some of which reached the book.

The fourth person without whom this book would not have been written is Emma Ashworth, herself a mother, a phenomenal maternity activist, a co-author and editor of some of AIMS' books and one-time editor of their journal. Emma took time out of her busy life to repeatedly read my early book drafts and critique with such perceptiveness what I was trying to say and the way I was saying it. This book is so much more readable and with references because of her. I am forever in her debt. Thank you.

I must also thank my readers who, in short order, read my book and gave insightful and detailed feedback. Your comments I found heart-warming and challenging by turns: I did my best with them. I hope you approve. It has been very humbling to have so many friends and colleagues endorse this book: usually you only get to hear such things when you are dead! Thank you to you all.

Thanks also to my talented daughter who designed the book cover, and to Airedale Mum Jo Whistler, who gave us permission to use and manipulate her joyous image.

Thank you to Kathryn Gutteridge, who wrote a most powerful foreword whose words ring out to challenge us all.

Meanwhile, Brenda, Olivia and Zara at Book Brilliance Publishing, in so many ways, are keeping this show on the road, editing, teaching and mentoring me through publication and beyond. Thank you is such a small word for a lot of work!

There is one midwife leader in Bradford who should have been in the text of this book but somehow none of the stories enabled this. Nevertheless, she very much needs to be present because without her, many of the successes – strategically but also for individual parents – would not have happened. Consultant Midwife Alison Brown, as she was at the time, is a woman and person-centred healthcare professional. As a midwife and midwifery leader, she is heart and soul 'with woman'. Her love and passion for the people she worked with, and the profession and service she was a member of, shone through all she said and did.

Alison has an innate ability to draw alongside people, to empathise in a way that enables people to feel they are heard and cared about – she was known in our circles as Granny Alison because it was like speaking to your granny. But alongside that was a determination, a focus and a vision to make Bradford's maternity care, in a very real and practical way, a woman and person-centred, quality service. I do not believe the Trust understands, acknowledges or appreciates the significance and importance of Alison Brown's work and vision because they let her go and dismantled much of what she put in place, along with the goodwill and relationships that she generated. Alison, for many parents, doulas, birth workers and activists, you remain our hero. Thank you.

This book would have not been written without the tribe of parents, birth workers, business people, community and civic leaders in Bradford and Airedale who in different ways were part of the network generating change. Although only one or two are named in the text, I had many allies: all the local MPs were supportive; there were local councillors who gave time and advice; the female community and city leaders networks were an essential community; as were the business advisors who helped us make a living whilst I also campaigned.

In addition, my thanks to the parents from whom I learnt so much and did some amazing stuff to bring about change, the doulas and doula networks, the La Leche League and other breastfeeding leaders who gave time so sacrificially, other birth workers who spread the love and worked for change. I hope you know who you are. I have huge respect for what you did and what you do.

In this age of bullying and malicious reporting of midwives to the NMC, I have been reluctant to name midwives but I want to salute the courage and determination of midwives who in different ways have worked for change from within the NHS and continue to do so.

I want to thank my midwives and those midwives and women who attended my births. With five children, I fear forgetting someone but I am sure you know who you are; however, a special shout out to Ann Devanny, Madge Boyle and Michelle Irving, as well as Tiffany Bisby and Jeanie Guest.

Finally, here and now I want to thank the independent midwives in West Yorkshire who were a rock-solid supportive community. I will always be indebted to you. I look forward to the day when the NHS recognises and respects fully the knowledge and professionalism of such midwives inside and outside the system.

I want to acknowledge and thank two organisations who have been particularly supportive of all my efforts over the years, and without whom, with their journals and databases, this book would not be so well referenced. AIMS and ARM, plus the committed volunteers who run them: thank you so much. Your work is essential and under-acknowledged.

At national and strategic levels, I have valued the conversations, time and kindness of a number of maternity leaders over the years who have illuminated complex issues and provided personal and strategic support. A special shout out to Cathy Warwick, Kathryn Gutteridge, the late Beverley Beech, Mary Newburn, Belinda Phipps, and Catherine Williams amongst others.

My husband and my family. There are really no words to express what it means to have the unconditional love and support of your family, and I know I am honoured and privileged to have it. These are the people who have plugged the gaps, tolerated my absences, made the meals, looked after the children. These are the people who have shared my dreams and helped them come true. These are the people who have held the broken pieces whilst I put myself back together again over and again. David and Judith Sharples. David Weston. Hannah, Bram, Tilly, Stan and Tom. Lynn Weston. Jane Wells. Thank you. I love you all.

About the Author

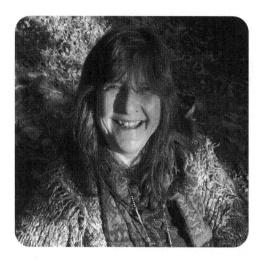

RUTH WESTON IS THE mother of five children, a social entrepreneur and an activist. After a degree in Theology and Church History, she studied at the Urban Theology Unit, Sheffield, where she learnt the practical grassroots organising and activism that put her theology to work.

In 1992, Ruth was appointed as Methodist Chaplain to Students at the University of Bradford and Bradford College. There she ran her first national campaign against student poverty and facilitated a student campaign against poor housing which yielded results still in place today.

After the birth of her first child, Ruth moved her community activism into the voluntary sector fulfilling a wide range of roles, including as School Governor at a school threatened with closure and as Chair of the support group for a local ex-offenders hostel.

It was only at the birth of her fourth child did she turn her phenomenal energy and focus on the maternity system. She built her birth pool business from a small local birth pool hire firm to a leading UK manufacturer of birthing pools and church baptistries. Ruth set up a small birth choices support group meeting in her home which became a regional and national network still functioning today through the Choices e-newletter.

Ruth featured in the *Desperate Midwives* documentary as the only woman to have a home water birth with an independent midwife. She featured in two other TV programmes and was interviewed for countless radio shows and newspaper articles.

Ruth chaired the stakeholder committee (then called the MSLC) for Bradford and Airedale Maternity, was part of a group that initiated Bradford Community Doula Scheme, and was a Breastfeeding peer supporter who helped set up a number of breastfeeding groups and advocated for peer support strategically.

She also took her campaign to improve maternity services to the national level, speaking at and chairing conferences, starting national campaigns, and writing to and meeting key figures in maternity.

Ruth is respected widely for her strategic and values-led thinking and her willingness to put her head above the parapet and speak out. Her story and the lessons we can all learn from them are written up in this book.

Keep in Touch!

Ways to work with Ruth:

- Workshops on Making Change Happen
- Course on How to make Change Happen
- Excellent Speaker and Conference Chair

Website: www.ruthweston.co.uk

Facebook page: www.facebook.com/profile.php?id=61556828767933

Facebook profile: www.facebook.com/RuthMWeston

Instagram: Ruth_Weston_Bornstroppy

LinkedIn: www.linkedin.com/in/ruthweston/

One Last Thing...

∾

Be a Dandelion

THE SPRING VERGES FILLED with the cheerful smiles of dandelions is a joy to the heart. Their cheerful yellow pompoms adorn walls and waste ground, and push up through cracks in the paving. They are ubiquitous, they are irradicable, they are everywhere.

As every gardener will tell you, the dandelion is one of the most effective pernicious weeds. It is almost impossible to eradicate the dandelion from your garden. Their taproots are deep and you must dig right down because if you leave one small piece of root in the ground, it will grow back from there. And if you drop one piece of root on the ground as you remove the offending plant - that too becomes a plant! So where you pulled up one dandelion, you can find a clump of dandelions growing a few weeks later. That is before you face the clouds of dandelion seeds floating on the wind from a thousand dandelion clocks.

Friends, we should be like dandelions: pernicious, ubiquitous, irradicable and everywhere. Our cheerful joyous smiles can be pulled up, but in our place, four more smiling flowers will return. The time for pioneers, for 'tall poppies', for boutique care teams and units is over, because like those unique shops and brands, they can be picked off one by one, closed down and destroyed. It is now time for the dandelion: a movement so cheerful, pernicious and vast that every attempt to destroy and close down results in a clump of cheerful flowers growing from its remnants.

Let us be dandelions. Maybe despised but nevertheless cheerful, pernicious, ubiquitous and everywhere.

And when the wind blows, our seeds will float far and wide, sharing the joy.

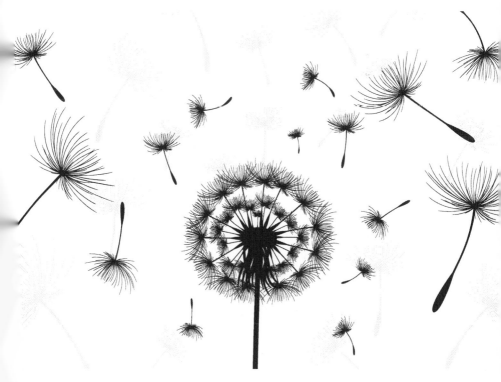